# In Search of the Good

**Basic Bioethics**
Arthur Caplan, editor

A complete list of the books in the Basic Bioethics series appears at the back of this book.

# In Search of the Good

A Life in Bioethics

Daniel Callahan

The MIT Press
Cambridge, Massachusetts
London, England

MIT Press books may be purchased at special quantity discounts for business or sales promotional use. For information, please email special_sales@mitpress.mit.edu or write to Special Sales Department, The MIT Press, 55 Hayward Street, Cambridge, MA 02142.

This book was set in Sabon by Toppan Best-set Premedia Limited, Hong Kong. Printed on recycled paper and bound in the United States of America.

Library of Congress Cataloging-in-Publication Data

Callahan, Daniel, 1930–
In search of the good : a life in bioethics / Daniel Callahan.
    p.   cm.—(Basic bioethics)
Includes index.
ISBN 978-0-262-01848-7 (hardcover : alk. paper)
1. Bioethics. 2. Callahan, Daniel, 1930– 3. Hastings Center. I. Title.
QH332.C35   2012
174.2—dc23
2012013229

10  9  8  7  6  5  4  3  2  1

For Sidney & Will & Betty
Without whom none of this would have been possible

For Thomas Murray & Eric Parens & Mary Crowley
Wonderful colleagues in my alleged retirement years

Jan Payne & Eva Topinková & Jeri Simek
To whom I brought bioethics and who gave me Czech friendship

# Contents

# Series Foreword

Glenn McGee and I developed the Basic Bioethics series and collaborated as series coeditors from 1998 to 2008. In Fall 2008 and Spring 2009 the series was reconstituted, with a new Editorial Board, under my sole editorship. I am pleased to present the thirty-fifth book in the series.

The Basic Bioethics series makes innovative works in bioethics available to a broad audience and introduces seminal scholarly manuscripts, state-of-the-art reference works, and textbooks. Topics engaged include the philosophy of medicine, advancing genetics and biotechnology, end-of-life care, health and social policy, and the empirical study of biomedical life. Interdisciplinary work is encouraged.

Arthur Caplan

*Basic Bioethics Series* Editorial Board
Joseph J. Fins
Rosamond Rhodes
Nadia N. Sawicki
Jan Helge Solbakk

# Preface

I have a peculiar trade. I think and write about bioethics, an updated and expansion of the ancient field of medical ethics. Exactly when I was first drawn in that direction is not clear. No doubt it had something to do with my early exposure to medicine. In the days prior to antibiotics, at the age of seven, I had infected lymph nodes in my groin. Time and again I was unwillingly carried to a hospital, an evil-smelling ether mask was put over my face, the nodes were lanced and drained, and then followed violent vomiting and weeks recuperating with painful daily bandage changes. It was hard to forget that first encounter with medicine and illness, which made me wary to this day of hospitals.

A more direct reason may have come later in my life, when my mother, responsible for the care of her sick Aunt Florence, got a call from her doctor to say that her leg was gangrenous and would have to be amputated to save her life. But then, he added, she would probably die on the operating table from the operation. What was my mother's choice? That was a good example of a term that was to become popular as bioethics moved along—a "hard choice"—which might better have been called an impossible choice. I have no recollection of my mother's decision.

Or it could have been some obstetricians talking about their delivery of a child, one of their great joys, yet one counterbalanced by women for whom an unwanted child was nothing less than a disaster. Or it could have been when I paid my mother a hospital visit as she was dying of cancer with only a few days left. She was still lucid and sitting up in bed. Her long-time doctor came to visit her and, to my astonishment, talked with my brother and me for about ten minutes and then left the room without looking at her or saying a single word to her. Was that the way a doctor should treat a patient?

One way or another, I was moving down a path that would lead me to be one of the founders of the field of bioethics and a co-founder of the Hastings Center, the first such research center in the world. Many date the origin of the field of bioethics to 1960, when the journalist Shana Alexander wrote an article for *Life* magazine about a committee in Seattle whose terrible task it was to decide which patients with failing kidneys would be put on a dialysis machine, which were still new and in short supply. They literally had to make life and death decisions case by case. Not much later a Harvard physician, Henry K. Beecher, brought down upon himself the wrath of his colleagues for blowing the whistle on medical researchers who didn't tell their patients they were part of dangerous research projects. The Nazi doctors of World War II were infamous for their lethal research on prisoners in death camps, and the revelation that something like that could be taking place in American medicine was hard to accept; the messenger was the one attacked.

Also during the 1960s, the contraceptive pill was invented, the first heart transplants were performed, intensive care units (ICUs) came into widespread use, complaints about the care of the dying grew as medical technology greatly expanded its capacity to keep very sick patients alive, and utopian dreams of genetic engineering were floating about. Medical progress was changing the definition of medicine, changing the conception of health, and changing the meaning of what it means to live a life. For someone educated as a philosopher, those were irresistible morsels.

I have often wondered how many Americans aim their life in one direction as they are growing up only to find that changes in themselves or the circumstances of their lives lead them in a very different direction, and how many find their lives leading to work or a field that did not even exist during their childhood or college years. My guess is: many.

I am a case study. Early in college I thought I would go into business, specifically into the transportation industry. I was enamored with trains and planes, and a college course I took was called "Trains, Planes, and Homing Pigeons." That romance did not last past my sophomore year. Much to my parent's bemusement, I began to fancy myself as an intellectual, drawn to capacious ideas and the mysteries of life. I decided to become a philosopher; I was told they thought about such things. Socrates was my model. As he learned, they may put you to death in the end for pushing hard questions on unwitting listeners, but that surely sounded more interesting than the economics of freight trains.

I went into philosophy with high hopes, came away disappointed with its academic embodiment, spent time as a magazine editor in New York, grew weary of that, and then wandered by way of writing a book on abortion into the ethical problems of medicine and biology. That was how I got into the field of "bioethics," a field I helped to invent, which is now named with a term that didn't even exist when I started down that path. Would it be possible to make use of my philosophical training on a wide and complicated range of ethical challenges posed by the stunning medical advances that emerged in the 1960s and promise along with others to continue for the indefinite future, as those challenges have?

Why not, I decided. At a 1968 Christmas party in Hastings-on-Hudson, New York, not far up the river from Manhattan, I recruited a neighbor and friend, psychiatrist and author Willard Gaylin, to help me start what came to be known as the Hastings Center. Just as I was being drawn to do research and to write well beyond the usual range of academic philosophy, Gaylin was similarly drawn to topics outside of professional psychiatry. I was Catholic by background and he was Jewish, but both of us had left religion behind us by that point in our lives. We liked to take on new topics we knew little about, enjoyed the play of ideas, and savored moving uninvited into other people's intellectual territory. I never wrote an article for a professional journal of philosophy, or even aspired to do so, and Will Gaylin had only written a few technical articles in his younger years for psychiatric journals. But we both made our way into the journals of many other fields, learning their folkways in the process. We liked to move around.

The attractions of the ethical issues of medicine and biology were many. They were immensely provocative, even dramatically so. They were new and relatively unexplored. They required cooperation among a wide range of disciplines, most notably medicine and biology, law and the social sciences, and philosophy and theology. And for someone trained in philosophy, there was a golden opportunity to move from ethical theory to clinical and policy application, an enticing combination.

All of us who lived through the 1960s and into the 1970s have our own selective memories of that era. Mine are not the drugs, sex, or politics of those days. I did smoke, unfiltered Pall Malls—and have the emphysema to prove it—but swore that once I kicked the habit I would never lecture or harass others to give it up, and I never did, reflecting a less than whole-hearted health zealotry. I suppose my six children suggest some level of sexual interest, and I religiously voted Democrat, but that was hardly radical stuff. Someone named Joan Baez sang nightly in a café just across the street from our house in Cambridge. I never set foot in the place and only later learned years later who she was. I did once take one of my children to demonstrate outside of the Pentagon (where I had once been stationed in the army) against the Vietnam War and spent an interesting evening at Columbia University to write about the antiwar campus riots there in 1968. That's about it for my counterculturalism. We did not, however, escape the parental agony of raising children in a time of too many drugs and too much alcohol and sex. We went to the police once too often in the middle of the night to recall that time with much nostalgia.

If I was not part of the counterculture, one feature of it caught my eye in passing, later to emerge in the context of bioethics. It was the tension between the hyperindividualism of the times and the parallel political movements. The hyperindividualism was personified by the hippies, an inchoate but roughly identifiable group that set about flouting convention, attacking authority in all guises, with an embrace of flagrant sexual promiscuity and drug use. The political movements by contrast focused on civil rights, solidarity in the face of racism, community organizing, and many efforts to establish communes. I was even then an emerging communitarian, and that latter political shift, no less a feature of the 1960s, was more congenial than the former.

But I suspected the hippie culture would win that culture war in the long run. The fast rise and equally fast decline of most communes in those days told the story—they were done in by middle-class young people who could not easily give up self-absorbed freedom in favor of the discipline and self-denial necessary for communal life and political impact. The emergence of a strong libertarian streak in the coming bioethics and the emergence of the Reagan market-saturated years was one of the results of the demise of the early communitarian stream of the 1960s.

What also caught my eye was a less-noted but strong feature of those times: an emerging ambivalence about technology. The post–World War II period had been marked by a great rush of money and enthusiasm for science and technology, symbolized perfectly by Vannevar Bush's characterization of science as "the endless frontier," by the beginning of a steady, even spectacular, rise in the annual budget of the National Institutes of Health (NIH) and by the excitement of the National Aeronautics and Space Administration (NASA) and space exploration.

But that enthusiasm came to be tempered by worries about the potential hazards of technology. The shadow of nuclear weapons and the possibility of a catastrophic war could not easily be ignored. The wonders of nuclear physics that gave us the bomb also opened the door to mutually assured destruction (MAD). The belief that the application of the latest and best in military technology guaranteed victory in Vietnam was one of the great illusions of that war. The new dreams about genetic engineering, promising the possibility of curing disease and improving human nature, came to be matched by visions of a suffocating *Brave New World*. Those wonderful ventilators, keeping us breathing on the brink of death, could also keep us going against all reason—even when our brains had been destroyed. Many years later, I wrote an article comparing two beloved national addictions: medical technology and the automobile. Both of them resist any kind of limits, but each of which if not checked—and they have so far have resisted any serious curbs—can create economic and environmental misery along the way.

Bioethics had a number of cultural roots. The ambivalence about technology was one of them. Another, a clear byproduct of the upheavals of the 1960s, was the suspicion of established institutions, which the discipline of medicine and the once-priestly role of the physician could not escape. Still another was the (slight) movement in my field, philosophy, away from academic theory to practical application, and for the humanities in general to be more socially "relevant," a term that often managed to irritate traditionalists while also not persuading the politically active that it was for real.

Although I was unaware of it at the time, I recall a study that demonstrated that the 1960s and 1970s were the glory days of the formation of research and policy institutions or "think tanks" as they came to be called (a phrase that all of us in them tended to hate). In creating the Hastings Center, we thought we were doing something rare and unusual. But as will become apparent more than once in this book, we were part of a larger movement that we could see only in retrospect. That kind of social phenomenon is always a little deflating for those who like to be thought of as bold pioneers. We were indeed just that, along with all the others.

If everything else is distilled out, what my career in bioethics comes down to is simple and enduring. It is an abiding fascination with the nature, scope, and validity of ethics as a part of human life, and a similarly strong interest in the ways that the scientific knowledge and technologies of medicine influence how we think about our health and mortality and shape the ways we live our lives. Along the way, that means thinking about human finitude; about illness, suffering, aging, and death; and about the place of health in our individual and collective lives. It no less requires a recasting of our ethical traditions and ways of thinking about them.

That agenda has been enough to fill a lifetime, and the aim of this book is to explain to myself and others how I have gone about this agenda. I will be 82 when this book is published—just the age, I have noted, when many of us turn from denying our advanced years to coyly beginning to brag about them. We are also, it is alleged, now the beneficiaries of the wisdom that comes with a long life. As much as I would like to believe it, I have never been convinced about the truth of that ancient conviction. But at the least, a long life does give one a good deal to write about, and that is not a bad second choice. If bits of wisdom slip into this book now and then, I can't help that. I may not know it when I see it.

Now, a word of warning. My chronology of events will sometimes be misleading, in part because I often cannot recall the sequence of ideas and perceptions as they germinated in my mind, often piecemeal over many years. Sometimes I think I have a great new idea—only to discover that I had said the same thing years before. Nor is there any necessary correlation between the events and issues I write about here and their importance to the field. I have chosen to write only about what in retrospect most interested me and shaped my thinking. Much, then, of the history of bioethics and even the Hastings Center over the past forty-three years will be missing altogether. And although an aim of this memoir is to show how at least one person trained in philosophy has come to think about the discipline, this is not a book about recent moral philosophy, but instead about some ways, often idiosyncratically, in which I have tried to digest it and make use of it in many nontraditional and nondisciplinary ways.

I came to think that trying to understand how medical progress actually affects our lives is the necessary first step in devising ethical solutions to the conundrums it throws upon us. In the end, I wanted to write in a way I enjoyed, not worrying about the scholarly niceties that I have felt necessary to attend to in most of my other books. I have tried to put Dr. Gradgrind behind me and have eschewed all but unavoidable gravitas. As my wife and I, who often took evening walks to discuss our writing—on death, suffering, dementia, evil, and the like—used to say, "Some couples have all the fun."

# Acknowledgments

Overcoming my skepticism, Mary Crowley urged me to write this memoir and helped me make it better. Will Gaylin, who knows all too much about me and the Center, brought his recollections to bear, as well as the sharp eye of a fellow writer. Renée Fox, herself a long-time observer of bioethics, was an insightful reader, as was Jack McClatchey, my college roommate. Susan Gilbert, a skilled editor, polished my writing and help me eliminate repetition. My wife, Sidney, brought her memory of all those years to the manuscript, often telling me I had something not quite right in the history I recounted. That is probably still true.

# 1

# Laying the Foundations: 1930–1961

To have a career reflecting on ethics requires three skills: to know oneself, to understand the culture in which one's life and one's profession are embedded, and to have a working knowledge of the history and methods of the field. In the vein of knowing oneself, I must then know where I came from. That contention has a particular importance in my case. Although I left the Catholic Church and religion in my mid-thirties, many friends and critics believe they can spot their remnants in me just below the surface. If true, I am hardly embarrassed by it. If anything that background gave me insights and perspectives I would not have otherwise have.

The Washington, D.C., I grew up in was hot, humid, and boring, and I got off to a good start by being born on July 19, 1930, a day (my mother later said) that set the all-time heat record for the city: 106 degrees. The Georgetown of the later Kennedy years, expensive and burnished, was then a black slum, and there was still fog in the "foggy bottom" that eventually became the home of the State Department. It was a one-company town, but that company—the federal government—was exactly what today's conservatives would like to return to: small, unobtrusive, relatively powerless, a dull gray in tone. The president still could and did ride about in a single car, not a caravan. There were only two good restaurants: Hogate's on the Maine Avenue waterfront and Occidental on Pennsylvania Avenue. Every year I was taken to one of them.

The government was not the Washington of my family. We were the locals, the natives (and, if wealthy, the "cave dwellers")—those who ran the small businesses and made their money as much off one another as from the government. My mother's family, farmers in southern Maryland on the Potomac, went back to the Virginia of the seventeenth century, and a great-great-grandfather, William Thorn, was bridgekeeper of the Aqueduct Bridge (the predecessor of Washington's Key Bridge) during the 1850s and 1860s. Stories of the returning soldiers from the Civil War walking north across that bridge were part of our family's lore. My father's family started in Philadelphia in the mid-nineteenth century as immigrants from Ireland and moved to Washington late in that century. My father knew little of that early history and seemed not to care. From that gap, we deduced that his family was escaping the potato famine, an event unlikely to inspire nostalgic memories of the old country.

My own contribution to our family's historical memory was a conversation I had in 1948 with an 85-year-old neighbor in Chevy Chase. He described to me his grandfather's first-hand account of the British burning the capital in 1814. He was at that time 10 years old and his grandfather in his mid-80s (so you can see that the math works out). "We kids thought it was a great lark," his grandfather said, "watching the fires and running about in the melee." Now that story, I thought, was one to pass along to my children, though I had none at the time nor any particular interest in history. No less memorable was an exchange with Alice Roosevelt Longworth, Teddy Roosevelt's lively daughter, at a Washington dinner party many years later. "Do your children," she asked, "have ponies?" "No," I said. She responded, "Oh, I'm sorry to hear that. My father thought them important for me to have at the White House when I was growing up." Down the same street from where I lived in Chevy Chase was the only daughter of F. Scott Fitzgerald, Francis Scott Lanahan, whose father's neglected grave in Rockville my wife and I were to visit a few years later, just when his writing was finding a new audience. Fitzgerald's first book, *This Side of Paradise*, captured the unease he felt as an undergraduate at Princeton—a midwestern Irish Catholic in the empire of settled WASP ascendancy—just what I later felt at Yale.

My father, Vincent F. Callahan, Jr., was born in 1902 as the youngest of eleven children; he had no education beyond high school, but he was ambitious and managed to land a job as a reporter for the *Washington Herald* (the predecessor of the *Washington Post*) in the 1920s. He met my mother, Anita Hawkins (seven years older than he was), a secretary, while covering the District of Columbia government office. They were married in 1925, and two years later he temporarily left her to take a job in 1927 with radio station KDKA in Pittsburgh, one of the first. He was in on the ground floor of American radio, which had started only a few years earlier. It was not just a new commercial technology; for someone of my father's modest background it was a move into the opening years of a new era, the advent of the modern media age.

He came back from Pittsburgh to become the advertising manager for WRC and WMAL in Washington and, in later years, managed radio stations in New Orleans (WWL) and Boston (WBZ). Those were hard years for my mother, called the "most beautiful woman in Washington" in 1927 by the *Washington Herald*. She was too often left at home by an alcoholic husband whose greatest pleasure was playing poker with his male pals in a back room at the National Press Club. His often jokingly nasty and belittling remarks intimidated all of us, and it was years before I had confidence enough to verbally assert myself. I was always waiting for a put-down.

My father lost his radio jobs because of his drinking and aggressive style but managed to land on his feet when he became director of radio and newspaper publicity for the War Bond campaign in the 1940s, working for Secretary of the Treasury Henry Morgenthau. In 1942 we drove across the country to Hollywood so that he could recruit movie celebrities, and it was a thrill to meet Jack Benny, Hedy Lamar, and Jack Warner, among others.

My father eventually lost that job because of some kind of scandal, whispered about but never openly described. But with Robert Kiplinger—the Washington newsletter pioneer—as a mentor, he moved into publishing newsletters for business on gaining government contracts, and from there on it was smooth sailing. After he died in 1964, my mother—now out from under him—blossomed. She took up painting, was part of a White House ladies speaking club, and eventually married a sweet and dear lawyer, Dan Ring, the polar opposite of my father. She always felt that if he had worked harder and remained sober, my father could have become president of a major radio network. Possibly so.

## My Catholic Heritage

My parents were both Roman Catholics, from my mother's English side and my father's Irish side, and this is where I will begin my own story.

As I discovered when I moved to Boston many years later, to be a Catholic in Washington was very different from almost every other large American city. There were no religious ghettoes or ethnic neighborhoods of any kind (save for blacks). Everyone was mixed together: Jews, Catholics, and Protestants (the majority), and I had childhood friends from each group. A few years ago, talking with my friend, physician-author Sherwin Nuland, I said that I did not hear any anti-Semitic talk when I was growing up. He thought that was utterly implausible for that era, and that I must be in some kind of denial, but I still think my recollection was true. My father's emergent world of radio was more open to diversity than most of America.

My father was a not uncommon kind of Catholic in those days. For the most part, he did not go to church, but he wanted my brother and me educated as Catholics and expressed alarm many years later when my wavering faith began to show. Although I remained a virgin throughout my high school and college years—up until marriage, for that matter—he seemed to expect that I would experiment a bit and dropped hints about the use of contraceptives. As I had no inkling of how one found girls to use them with, my reaction was a baffled "What's up with him?" As far as I could make out, his many siblings were faithful Catholics, though I always wondered why the nine of them who married produced only seven children among them (though those were the years when many husbands and wives slept in separate beds or rooms). Only later did I learn that women born from 1900 to 1920—my mother's generation—had the fewest children per women in the twentieth century, and some 20 percent never married, a figure not reached again until recent years. My mother's Catholicism was different. She did go to church regularly and, on the surface, was a more serious Catholic than my father. Yet from time to time in her later years, she would voice some quiet skepticism about it all, but only in passing and in a cryptic way. I should have pressed her on that, but it did not seem appropriate for me to do so (though I now think, why not?).

I was sent to parochial schools in New Orleans and Washington and was taught by nuns. I have none of the hostile recollections of nuns that mark many Catholic memoirs, but then I have no fond recollections either. They were a tough-minded bunch, not at all averse to a bit of corporal punishment, from a whack with a ruler to a pinching of the ear.

I did not do well in the Washington parochial school, St. Thomas, which was across the street from the Wardman-Park Hotel. I paid too much attention to the girls and could not sit still, I was told—surely an accurate description. I am certain that these days I would be diagnosed as a troubled hyperactive kid and put on drugs, but in those days there was an alternative: military school.

Beginning with the seventh grade, I was sent to St. John's College (actually a high school) at Thomas Circle in Washington and spent the next five years in uniform and with daily marching. The teachers, all male, were members of the LaSalle Christian Brothers order, and they were a nice bunch, fanatical neither about their religion nor about education. We took a fine range of courses, Latin and French, English, biology, chemistry and physics, religion and history—but all taught in a low-key way with little, if any, homework. The military side was no less low key. We learned how to march and to hold (but not shoot) a gun. I was not a military star—I was one of the few seniors in my school not made an officer. When I went into the army later on, I applied for and was turned down for officer candidate school, lacking leadership potential. It was a sweet pleasure later to be chosen as one of 200 outstanding young leaders by *Time* magazine in 1975, right up there with Pete Dawkins the West Point football All-American star and Rhodes Scholar, who had everything I didn't. My basketball hero, Bill Bradley, was also in the group, as was my later friend Richard Lamm, who became governor of Colorado and was, along with me, notorious for suggesting that limits might have to be set on health care for the elderly.

I was only a fair to middling high school student, and my parents, though supportive, were not the least pushy. My mother once said, in fact, that she did not think I was especially smart. The comment did not bother me all that much because that was my view of myself also. But a bit of envy of Jewish kids did cross my mind. I had been told that their mothers extravagantly praised them, told them they were geniuses, and expected them to do great things with their lives. I got no such flattery. But two things of importance happened in high school. On land I began to take religion seriously, even becoming a bit pious, and in the water I became a local swimming star.

I can't say exactly why religion became important to me. Most important was probably what can be called a burgeoning religious experience, that of a sense of awe and transcendence at Mass and during other religious devotions. I was moved, and when that happens to people they take a different stance toward religion: it becomes something more than a set of beliefs or an act of faith.

## Swimming: Opening the Way to the Rest of My Life

My swimming was almost as important as religion for my early life. Not big enough for football, tall enough for basketball, or talented enough for baseball, I cast about for another sport, settling on long-distance swimming, from 200 to 1,500 meters. I am not sure swimming does much to improve one's character, but the boring and tiring practice does reward perseverance. The distance events I swam also rewarded a willingness to put up with pain, a useful trait for later in life. Displaying some of the entrepreneurial skills that would serve me well in later years when I helped found the Hastings Center, I talked St. John's into forming a swimming team and got myself elected as both captain and coach. I won a number of Washington championships and—best of all—won an annual three-mile race in the Potomac River at the Key Bridge in 1948. That was the last such race in the river (canceled because of pollution) and I am therefore to this day the reigning District of Columbia long-distance swimming champion. It is surely the only permanent title I will ever hold, and I selfishly hope that the race is never started again.

But the pleasure of swimming turned out to be the less important reason for its importance in my life. That point is that it led me to Yale, which at that time had the leading swimming team in the world: long undefeated and populated by world-record breakers in just about every event, but particularly mine. I have always had some affection for affirmative action programs, if only because I was a beneficiary of one in 1948. I did poorly on my SATs (mid-600s verbally and 375 in math!), came from a third-tier high school, and had good grades only in my senior year. I was not exactly competitive with those white-shoe kids from Andover and Exeter, who—myth had it—had taken courses in Assyrian literature, astrophysics, and Hegel. But I was a swimmer, which Yale wanted, smart or not, and I was Catholic. Next to Jews, Yale had traditionally disliked Catholics only slightly less, but it now appeared to be making amends. I was accepted, and on my way to the rest of my life.

My teachers at St. John's were ambivalent about my acceptance at Yale. They were proud that one of their own had made it to an Ivy League school (which had happened only once before, years earlier). They were also openly fearful that I "would lose my faith," and some Catholic schools would not even forward transcripts to such schools. Their vision of Yale and its kind was that of sinkholes of atheism and agnosticism, snobbish, antireligious, thoroughly materialistic, and shot through with Communist ideas. William F. Buckley, Jr.—not a classmate but at Yale during my time, and my Spanish examiner—was later to make his name with *God and Man at Yale*, an attack on the secularism and left-leaning bent of the faculty. He made an outsized student reputation at Yale, but we Catholics were mainly interested in how he crashed through the Protestant culture barrier: one of our own had made it. Years later, as he often did with his critics, he invited my wife and me for an evening sail after I wrote an article critical of him, and well after that I appeared on his TV show *Firing Line*.

My high school teachers were probably right about my losing the faith, but only in the long run. I did eventually lose it, though I am not sure how much Yale had to do with that, or even my later time at Harvard. For my first three years at Yale, I was mainly a swimmer, going to the ornate Payne Whitney gym at least once and sometimes twice a day. I was not, however, a great swimmer, especially when up against Olympians and world-record holders in my events. But I did learn how to be a loser and, more important, how to focus my energy on working or competing in only those activities that I liked for their own sake, win or lose. I came to care about only my own times—how well was I competing against myself—not whether I won (just once) or lost (every other time) a race.

## Coming Up Out of the Water and into Philosophy

I retired from swimming at the end of my junior year. My last Yale meet was against Harvard, in Cambridge. I was put in the 440-yard freestyle in place of the Yale world-record holders, and when my name was announced, the 2,000 spectators booed. They had not come to see me, but our stars. Well, I would show them! I did not; I came in last. That was not the final blow to my swimming ego, however, which came when a 12-year-old beat me in a Washington summer championship meet. There is losing and there is *losing*, and that was *losing*. I got out of the pool, dried off, and asked myself whether my swimming career was at an end. "What else is going on at Yale?" I thought.

I was, in a way, lucky to still be there. During my freshman year, juggling swimming and a part-time job in one of the colleges, I got poor grades and actually failed biology. I was about to flunk out. My freshman advisor went to my biology professor, George Baitsell, saying that the only thing that would save me would be a change in my grade. Professor Baitsell said, "Fine; no problem," and he moved me from an F to a D on the spot, and that did it. In light of my later career in bioethics, requiring I know something about biology and medicine, that was not an auspicious start. But it was all the formal biological science I ever had after high school. It was a delicious pleasure, some twenty-five years later, to give a named lecture in the same classroom where I had failed the biology course. You can fool some of the people some of the time. And if I proved to be no good at science, I found myself doing much better in writing and the humanities.

A more important part of my education was to take part in an early experimental interdisciplinary program mixing literature, history, and psychology. The courses I took added up to no coherent whole, but they were to serve later as a powerful antidote to the analytic philosophy I was to receive at Harvard. The world was richer than our language and full of realities other than concepts and logical entailments. Paul Desjardins, an older Catholic graduate student getting a Ph.D. in philosophy at Yale and writing a dissertation on the Socratic dialogues, befriended me. He was one of the world's great talkers, never publishing a word over a long career as a professor at Haverford College, and a master of the Socratic method in his work with students.

He once made an indelible impression upon me when, after he'd taken his laundry to a Chinese laundry, he asked me, "How did I do?" I did not understand the question, so he clarified it: "I mean how did I do in dealing with my Chinese laundry man? How should someone who is a Yale instructor treat someone who does his laundry? Should it be different from the way I treat my Italian barber?" I had no answer to such questions then, but they helped fix in my mind an important point about ethics, which begins at the borderline of etiquette and with the seemingly trivial details of daily life.

Another event of importance was a course on Thomas Aquinas, taught by an unusual (for Yale) visiting professor, prominent Jesuit John Courtney Murray. A friend of Clare Booth Luce, and well known in some fashionable circles, he was—though I did not know it at the time— engaged in a great struggle to get the Church to accept the notion of freedom of religion and life in a pluralistic society. He had been silenced on occasion but was finally able to make his mark at the Second Vatican Council in the 1960s. He was a tall and imposing figure, somewhat distant, and no doubt preoccupied at the time in doctrinal debates with the Vatican that never reached lay ears. His course was rather routine, but at least I had a chance to read Aquinas and to learn about natural law theory, about which I later heard nothing at all at Harvard. His course, plus Paul's influence, was sufficient to convince me that I should go for a Ph.D. in philosophy.

Before I could do that I had to serve in the army, as the Korean War was winding down, as a volunteer in the counterintelligence corps (CIC) and, along the way, to get married and complete an M.A. in philosophy at Georgetown. How could I do all that while in the army? In one of the oddest of military careers, I was assigned not to Korea, but to the Pentagon in Washington. And because those in the CIC worked in civilian clothes and received a living allowance for off-base housing, I promptly moved back in with my parents, took a bus to the Pentagon each night, and used the housing allowance to begin my studies at Georgetown.

There is not much to say about my time in the Pentagon—looking at night for security violations such as open safes, classified documents lying on desks, and other heavy-duty threats to national security. More interesting was a task assigned to our unit: investigating the charge of Senator Joseph McCarthy about Communists or fellow travelers in the army. That was a big mistake on his part. He looked foolish and the beginning of his end came into sight. I spoke with the Senator once. When not on stage, he came across as a quiet and assuming man. "Uncle Joe" Stalin apparently made the same impression on strangers, just before he ordered their execution.

## Sidney: My "Bluestocking" Wife

I was married in Washington in 1954, my second year in the army. I was 24, and my new wife, Sidney, was 21. Born in Washington also, but with deeper Alabama roots, she had gone to a girl's school, Holton-Arms, which was the female prep school equivalent of St. Alban's, Landon, and Sidwell Friends—a social grouping well above my lower-middle class-mates at St. Johns. A convert to Catholicism—only partially because of me after moving through a variety of Protestant churches—and the daughter of a career naval officer, she was in her junior year at Bryn Mawr when we married, graduating in 1955, as she put it, "magna cum baby."

We were well matched. Sidney had made her mark with her parents as a teenager by begging off from playing bridge, asking to be let alone so she could read. Strange behavior for a well-bred southern girl. A few of my Yale classmates warned me about marrying an intellectual ("blue-stocking") woman. I was planning to go into philosophy, not a career that would commend me to her father. Even my parents, though they tried, could not extract from me a clear answer to a sensible parental question: just what is philosophy? Even now I doubt that I could give a persuasive answer to that question. The comic book version goes something like this, and it's not too far off: it has something or other to do with truth; whether there is a real world outside of our sense perceptions; and if all men are mortal, and I am a man, whether I am mortal; and whether there is any way to know what goes on in the minds of other persons. As my son John noted at my 1996 retirement dinner, the really remarkable thing is that "people actually get paid to think about such questions."

My religious development now moved into a new stage. I now had a wife who shared my Catholicism and, even more, my kind of Catholi-cism. We were both readers of *Commonweal*, a lay-edited liberal weekly (whose staff I would later join), fervent Democrats, and followers of Dorothy Day and the Catholic worker movement, aiming to live and work in poverty. A critical book for us was called *Be Not Solicitous*. Its theme was that the serious Christian should give no thought to the future, eschewing insurance and other sources of security and, above all, accept-ing all the children God sent. It projected a life radically open to the future, full of risk but full of joy as well. That phase did not last long, but I brought some lingering vestiges of that spirit to the founding of the

Hastings Center at age 39, with six children, a wife working to get her Ph.D., and no job.

I was aiming for an academic life after my degree, and my wife, eager for us to have many children, wanted six of them by age 30 and a Ph.D. by 35 (it actually took her until age 47 to get the degree, which was partly my fault, but we had the six children by the time she was 32). We had no materialistic ambitions, but we did want to go to the best schools and do all we could for our children. Although it was true that our desire for children was inspired by our Catholicism (left-wing) branch, demography and the zeitgeist plays tricks on patterns on cycles of procreation. My wife was born in 1933; women born in this year had more children than any other year in the twentieth century, an average of 3.8. We were not quite as procreationally radical as we thought. And when I worked at the Population Council some years later, I discovered that most of the senior scientists and researchers at that wholly secular family planning and population control organization had three or four children. I could not help thinking often of my father's family, with its grand total of seven offspring, but then my parents' generation had married during the Depression years, which saw a great drop in birth rates for Catholics and everyone else.

## Preparing to Be an Academic Philosopher

While still a commuting soldier, I entered an M.A. program in philosophy at Georgetown University in 1954. It was altogether fitting that the building that housed the philosophy department had earlier been the old Georgetown Hospital, where I been born. In the fall of 1956, out of the army and with an M.A. and one child, I entered the Ph.D. program in philosophy at Harvard. Why Harvard? The Yale department, considered the best at the time, turned me down. I recalled liking the Harvard campus from my swimming meet there—not what could be called a very good reason for choosing a graduate program, and one about whose faculty and reputation I knew nothing. But the Harvard philosophy department took me, and that was a good enough reason.

There had ever been, I discovered, only been a handful of Catholics in that department, and I was a curiosity. I found it a strange and gradually distasteful department, not at all fitting my romantic picture of philosophy. Historian Bruce Kuklick published a book in 1977, *The Rise of American Philosophy*, which despite the title was actually a history of the Harvard philosophy department. His thesis was illuminating and was being acted out before my eyes. In the nineteenth and early twentieth centuries, there was no tight discipline of philosophy. Apart from students, the audience of philosophers was assumed to be the general public, not other philosophers, and with the possible exception of Charles Sanders Peirce (the first pragmatist), William James, George Santayana, and Josiah Royce—among others—wrote essays and books accessible to the educated and filled with references to history, literature, religion, and the classics.

But as Kuklick showed, by the 1940s philosophy was becoming a narrow, more technical academic discipline, increasingly directed toward other philosophers. As he put it, "During the same period in which philosophy became a profession [the 1930s], political and social theorizing continued to occupy a minor place . . . when narrow professionals turned to their scholarship, they thought of their work as a game. For a few, professional philosophy had become a way, not of confronting the problem of existence, but of avoiding it." That is harsh, but not far from the professional philosophy to which I was introduced many decades later, including the word "game."

That later kind of department was the one I entered. By then it also had an added twist. It was dominated by the kind of philosophy fostered at Oxford and Cambridge, focusing on conceptual and linguistic analysis. Willard Van Orman Quine, a distinguished logician and analytic philosopher, was the dominant figure. I had no idea beforehand of the flavor or the substance of the department, and it was unsettling. I had been drawn to philosophy by the example of Socrates, who went about Athens asking large and questions in the Agora and getting his hemlock comeuppance for doing so. The message I got at Harvard was, in effect, "Hey kid, we don't do that kind of thing any more." Our introduction to the history of philosophy (which unreconstructed analytic philosophers dismissed as "not philosophy" at all) moved from Plato and Aristotle (both only lightly touched upon) to Kant and the British empiricists in the eighteenth century, and from there another 200 or so years to twentieth-century Oxford philosopher J. L. Austin. We skipped, among other philosophers, Thomas Aquinas and the Medievals, Hegel and the German idealists, Adam Smith, Karl Marx and Nietzsche, just about all political philosophy, Heidegger, and Sartre and the existentialists.

We did learn a good deal about utilitarianism, Kant, and deontology, and we were introduced to the leading analytic philosophers of the day, almost all of whom were nurtured at Oxford or Cambridge: G. E. Moore, Bertrand Russell, Ludwig Wittgenstein, and A. J. Ayer. The characteristic feature of all of them was a focus on concepts and language, analyzed in great detail and heavily shadowed by the dominance of science and the earlier logical positivists. A. J. Ayer achieved a wide reputation with his 1936 book *Language, Truth, and Logic*, which touted the "verification principle," the idea that the only meaningful ideas were those open to scientific verification. To say that the Mona Lisa was a great painting, or that it was good not to tell lies, is no more than to express my feelings, called "emotivism." The verification principle at one stroke threw ethics, aesthetics, and religion into the dustbin of history, amounting to no more than mere scientifically unverifiable emotional expressions.

G. E. Moore's formulation of the "naturalistic fallacy" complemented Ayer by contending that there is a fundamental divide between facts and values and that moral rules and principles could not be derived from factual knowledge: an ought cannot be derived from an is. Of course, one response is to note that "is" is all there is in the world, and if ethics cannot be developed from that it is hard to see how it can be justified at all. But that was just what many of the analytic philosophers of that era actually believed. Although emotivism and the Ayer-like positivism did not have a long intellectual life, I could see their lingering influence on many of the doctors I encountered later in my work at the Hastings Center in the 1970s. They believed that science was the only source of real knowledge and that ethics was nothing more than emotion-driven opinion, with religion lurking just below the surface.

As for the philosophers of that postwar era, British philosopher Mary Midgely noted that the one thing they did not go near was the inner life of humans, neither their own nor anyone else's. Not once did I hear anything said in or out of the classroom about how we should live our lives, that most ancient of all ethical quests. It is worth noting that some of the leading Oxbridge women philosophers of that era—Phillipa Foote,

Iris Murdoch, Elizabeth Anscombe, and Midgely—were critical of that omission among their male counterparts.

We were warned in the philosophy department not to go near Professor John Wild, who taught a course on existentialism. To show an interest in that sort of conceptually muddy stuff (as bad as Hegel) was a professional kiss of death. Philosophy, one distinguished logician told me, was best thought of as a kind of game, technical and intricate, that only a few highly educated—and of course very smart—people liked to play. If one asked, "What is the meaning of life?" the not-quite-joking answer was, "Life has no meaning; only propositions have meaning."

## Ethics from the Perspective of an Ideal Observer

My worst experience was with my professor of moral philosophy, Roderick Firth, who taught the main course in the subject and held the view that the best perspective on ethical truth was that of an "ideal observer," detached, disinterested, and all-knowing; that was the way to know right from wrong. How one became such an observer was, perhaps not inexplicably, left unexplained. Each year, the various professors would devote an evening to talk about their own philosophical positions, and Professor Firth once talked about his ideal observer theory. Having heard that he was a Quaker, I asked him how he related the moral values of Quakerism, such as its pacifism, to moral philosophy. He was not pleased with the question, stiffly responding, "I don't think that is an appropriate question for this evening Mr. Callahan. Perhaps you should visit me during office hours." He then abruptly turned away and said to the audience, "Next question?" A few of my fellow students defended his answer by saying, "But that was a religious, not a philosophical question." Oh.

At that moment, I think the seed was planted that would lead me to eventually conclude that I did not want to spend the rest of my life in such academic company, with philosophy considered to be a kind of game and with an almost total bifurcation of academic ethics and one's personal moral life. I found that a great way to start an argument with a philosopher (and it's good to this very day) was to contend that one had to be a good person to think well about ethics. Nonsense, I was invariably told: it is only the quality of one's arguments that counts, and that is a function of one's smarts, not one's moral sensibilities, whatever they might be.

It was probably no accident that the two of my later most prominent classmates, writer Susan Sontag and civil rights leader Robert Moses, were dropouts. I found it a cold and competitive department; putting one's fellow students down was not infrequent. Only three of the seventeen students who started in my year ever got their degree; most of the others faded away, bored and disappointed. The next generation of professors, led by John Rawls and Robert Nozik, were a more genial group (or so I've been told), and the generation of young philosophers who founded the journal *Philosophy and Public Affairs* were surely different (though that journal too seemed to be aimed at other philosophers).

When later asked what I learned in my years at Harvard, it took me a while to find an answer: I learned how to ask, with the proper Oxford snarl, "But what do you *mean* when you say something is 'good'?"—an all-purpose, deliberately intimidating question when talking about ethics. I should add that I was anything but a great student, failing my prelims twice, the German exam twice as well, and having my dissertation twice rejected. I barely made it out of there. I was thus greatly pleased when, in 2006, the Harvard Graduate School of Arts and Sciences, the home of the philosophy department, awarded me its Centennial Medal.

Fortunately, there was more to Harvard than the philosophy department. By the end of our time there, we were up to three children, all boys. We lived for a time in a Harvard-owned house featuring gaps in the floor boards, a balky coal furnace that required pampering in the middle of the night, and a sink in which the water froze when the temperature dipped below zero degrees outside—a frequent event. A Harvard maintenance man told my wife that even at $35 rent a month, "It isn't worth it, lady." But, lacking money, we were taking the ideal of poverty seriously. That did us little good with our seriously poor Cambridge neighbors who, bothered by our noisy boys, complained about "you Harvard people." They saw what was less obvious to us, that poor Harvard graduate students were not the same as poor real people.

Yet the Harvard and Cambridge of those days were marked by genteel shabbiness. Neither undergraduates nor graduate students ate out much, and the one decent restaurant, Chez Dreyfus, was known as the place you took your visiting parents. During that time, we also began getting lectures from our classmates, save for the Mormons, about the virtues of family planning. My wife's response was to say that "the Pope gives us a gold star for every baby," which she knew some of them were naïvely prepared to believe.

We lost a baby, Thomas, at forty-two days to crib death during our last year at Harvard and on my wife's birthday, March 6. A granddaughter who now lives with us, and whose mother died in childbirth, was also born on March 6. Sudden infant death syndrome (SIDS) has to this day not been given a definitive cause, and its sudden and unexpected appearance with a dead baby in a crib left my Sidney for years wondering if she was somehow at fault. It is possible, we found, to feel guilty about something one had not caused, all reason to the contrary. Many doctors, I learned later, feel that way when a patient of theirs dies. Could they have possibly done more?

## An Antidote to Analytic Philosophy: Discovering Culture

By the late 1950s, I had begun writing for *Commonweal*. I had written the editor out of the blue, telling him what a smart fellow I was—Harvard pedigree, no less—offering to review books and noting that I had taken much English literature at Yale. That was a bit of an exaggeration, but I had learned at Yale that it was better to oversell than undersell. My first assignment was to review a book by the distinguished literary critic Hugh Kenner, whose theories I did not understand, and I had never read the books and authors he cited. Actually, to say I "did not understand" what I was reading puts the matter with less than precision: I had no idea at all what he was talking about, not a clue. That lacuna was solved by recruiting a friend getting a degree in English to read the book and to tutor me about what to say. That was my inauspicious, slightly shady start, and I began writing regularly for the magazine. Later, I sometimes even knew what I was talking about.

I soon became a minor name in Catholic intellectual circles at Harvard and elsewhere. My interest in religion led me to make friends at the Divinity School and to put together an ecumenical discussion group, one of the first in the country. Harvey Cox, Michael Novak, and John T. Noonan were among the young up-and-comers at Harvard during those years, and out of that group came my first book, *Christianity Divided* (1961), one of the first ecumenical collections of Protestant and Catholic essays. Shortly thereafter, I was asked to serve as an assistant to Christopher Dawson, an historian of religion and culture and the first holder of the Chauncey Stillman chair in Roman Catholic Studies at the Divinity School. His writings focused on the role of religion, particularly Christianity, as a necessary foundation for viable cultures.

Dawson was an odd but interesting person. He once said to me that "the world ended when the queen died," meaning Queen Victoria. He was about as old-fashioned and rooted in the past as that statement might suggest, but a lucid and interesting historian. He graduated from Oxford prior to World War I and saw many of his friends and classmates killed in the war. He never taught, just wrote, and Harvard was his first and only academic appointment.

I was brought in because his teaching style was soporific—even mind-numbing. He simply read from manuscripts in a low monotone voice that could hardly be heard, even around a seminar table. When asked questions, he usually answered them with some mumbled words at most, and sometimes just one word. "Did the Reformation have some economic roots?" he was once asked. He was silent, pondering for about a minute, and then answered, "Yes." Just yes. It was my job, for all four of his students, to liven things up, to elaborate on his monosyllables, to Americanize his seminar. I knew nothing whatever about the history of religion, much less its place in different cultures, but somehow he thought that I did and I scrambled every day to skim history books and find out what he was talking about. Don't ask me now who Felicite de Lamennais was, as I held on to such information for no more than a day. But my experience with Dawson instilled in me an interest in the shaping force of culture, which I thereafter brought into all my writing.

I might add that the Divinity School was treated with maximum scorn in the philosophy department, as in most of the university. Harry Levin, a noted English professor, once said that Divinity Avenue began with biology laboratories but ended with the desert that was the Divinity School. The small, old-fashioned building that housed the Divinity School was soon surrounded by large, modern science classrooms and laboratories, saying something about the move away from religion to science as the successor king of the mountain.

## George Berkeley: Language and Ethics

I thought that the theologians had all the interesting questions about life, but no methodology of any great value in answering them, and that the philosophers had great methodologies to answer uninteresting questions. Neither judgment was quite true—and many scientists thought that their way of thinking was better than both of them—but the contrast between those two distant worlds was enormous. Aiming to stay out of trouble, I never mentioned in the philosophy department that I was moonlighting in *that* place, a far worse offense even than taking the existentialism course.

I finished out my days at Harvard by writing my dissertation on eighteenth-century Irish-English bishop and philosopher George Berkeley. He was historically famous for his belief that to be is either to perceive or to be perceived—*esse est percipi aut percipere*. I was not drawn to that extraordinarily implausible view, but he had more to say than that. Writing in his dialogue, the *Alciphron,* he held that the language of religion and ethics should be understood as moving us to feeling and action, not describing the world. That was an adventurous view in his day, at a time when it was thought, especially by John Locke, that language was primarily used to name objects. Berkeley was in effect a precursor to Ludwig Wittgenstein, who famously said, "Don't look to the meaning but to the uses of a word." The topic was suggested to me by Henry Aiken, the other professor of moral philosophy. It was a fortuitous choice. Berkeley wrote the *Alciphron* in 1730, having come to Rhode Island to start a college in Bermuda under the mistaken belief that it was an island convenient to the entire eastern seaboard. He never found the money to do that, but he left for me two models: a masterfully clear and elegant writing style and, in his life, a good person, beloved and revered. His house, outside of Providence, is still standing.

## Deriding Wisdom

Nonetheless, if my life in the philosophy department was unsatisfactory, some attitudes I developed at Harvard have endured. One of them is an abiding suspicion of the naïve view that clean and pure reason is the answer to everything, a view that is only a shade removed from a belief that science is the only reliable source of knowledge. Philosophy can do some mopping up around the edges (as Quine himself seems to have held), but that is about all.

While not quite dead, the idea that philosophy is meant to be a search for wisdom had come upon hard times. As someone who has always been drawn to literature, history, and the social sciences, and at one time to religion, I had effectively been inoculated against hard-core, antiseptic rationalism. That is not the way human life is experienced or lived, even by the rationalists themselves when off duty. As my wife once observed after a long meeting with a leading group of young moral philosophers, the editors of *Philosophy and Public Affairs*—many of whom she got to know well outside of the conference room—"They talk about ethics one way around the conference table and very differently about it in their personal lives." The most glaring deficiency in the moral philosophy of the 1940s and 1950s was a total absence of any interest in how we should live and shape our lives. "Virtue theory" had a number of theological adherents but few in philosophy. There has been some revival of that tradition since then.

If I was put off by the pretense of rationalism, I was no less alienated from the aggressive secularism that went with it. The hostility to religion was pervasive, which although excessive was perhaps understandable for many escapees from orthodox Judaism and conservative Protestantism. Less understandable was a disinterest in even trying to understand religion. Susan Sontag was an exception. She once asked me to talk at length with her about my religious beliefs. The closest anyone else got was when an instructor in logic asked me why Catholics wore their overcoats in church rather than hang them up as in Protestant churches. Well, that was a stumper and to this day I have no good answer to that probing question. Maybe the Catholic churches are just colder. Who knows?

**Twin Brothers: Dogmatic Religion and Dogmatic Secularism**

Yet if "dogmatic religion," as it was often called, had been put harshly aside, dogmatism of a different kind had not been. The secularism was as rigid in its beliefs and mores as the most dogma-bound Roman Catholicism, only less aware of its own kind. Those believers in freedom and tolerance had little tolerance for people outside of their circle. But there was something worse that became apparent from time to time. It was an inflated sense of what personal freedom meant in the moral sphere for secular true believers: that the only binding moral obligations are those voluntarily chosen, not those thrust upon us by life in common with others.

The first sign of that I noticed was when I was a freshman advisor at Harvard and my wife and I took in the destitute wife (and her child) of an older advisee of mine who had abandoned her. To my astonishment, I was actually berated by some of my colleagues in the writing program for doing that. It was, they said, not part of the advisor role, not part of the contract, and just plain out of place. It was an attitude I saw played out again in different ethical contexts, and it reappeared in the mid-1990s when we brought home to live with us one of my sons (an impecunious screen writer) and his newborn daughter, whose mother had died in childbirth. Some people said we were saintly for doing that in our mid-60s, but others were unimpressed. What we had done was not part of the parent-child contract, thus making it inexplicable: the statute of limitations on parental responsibility had long ago run out. Why in the world did we do that? But then there were those who understood well what we had done: you don't have to be a saint to welcome back home children who have no money or other home. What else is one supposed to do?

Thousands of parents have had to do that lately because of the recession (more than six million grandparents are primary caretakers of their grandchildren). Social contract theories of ethics going back to Thomas Hobbes hold that societies are glued together by our mutual understanding that the common welfare requires accepting law, moral rules, and government oversight. I would add that a moral life requires that we accept and endure many burdens in life that are thrust upon us by accident, outside of the social contract that holds the larger society together. John F. Kennedy once memorably said that to have children is to be "hostage to fortune." True enough, but no less true of many other features of a life lived in common with others.

I have related here the first stage of my life, from my birth through my early 30s, encompassing my family history and formal education. Although I did not know it at the time, I was laying the foundation for my later work in bioethics. Although it surely made some difference, I am at a loss in understanding exactly how it did so. I cannot recall much at all about my religious training, other than to say that it was of a conventional kind for a Catholic child: be virtuous, do good, love thy neighbor, feed the poor, and visit the sick. We were expected to marry (cohabitation was unheard of), to hold off from sex until after that event, and then to have children. One was expected to do well economically but not to aspire to great wealth or a fast-track life. Though the term was not in use in those days, it seems fair to say that the model lifestyle was "laid back": not too ambitious or materialistic, and at all times nice, not pushy. The kind of person you are is what counted in the long run. That was a good legacy from my youth.

I can recall no mention whatsoever of some ethical issues that would preoccupy me later for a time: contraception and abortion, welfare policy, just warfare, and the eradication of racism. But many decades after I left both the church and religion, many people over the years have told me that my background Catholicism still shows in many ways. At the least it gave me the helpful advantage of being an outsider in the Protestant cultures of Yale and Harvard, both cultures that had become heavily secularized in the academic departments. At Harvard there was the double whammy of Protestants and secular Jews (who had their own problems with the Protestant culture), both of whom were suspicious of Catholicism. But that background forced me to see the larger society and the smaller academic world from a different angle.

## What Ethics Requires

Thanks to my Harvard education in moral philosophy, I came to understand that good work in ethics requires care and diligence. And that combination, together with my earlier swimming days, has served me well. I don't think of myself as a class-A workaholic (I have never once in my professional life stayed up late at night to meet a deadline), but most other people probably think of me that way, unaware of my long-term infatuation with movies and, of late, a garden (Voltaire had a point). But substantively, it was a poor education for a life of work in ethics. Too many major figures and important ideas were skipped and often scorned. The not-so-hidden belief that philosophy really began only with the Oxbridge analytic movement (but grandfathering in Locke, Kant, and the eighteenth-century British empiricists), clearing up centuries of confusion and muddled language, closed rather than opened the mind. The belief in objective, detached, and impersonal rationality was simply naïve, but seductively so.

The whole idea of shaping and living a moral life that is open to the widest range of human experience had been abandoned at the altar of narrowly focused disciplinary goals and a view of ethics deprived of interest in the ancient Greek admonition to "know thyself," much less the admonition that I would add, "know thy culture (starting with your own)." As an editor of the distinguished British journal *Philosophy* once said scornfully of another philosopher admired by my colleague Willard Gaylin, "He was a very good philosopher until he got interested in '*wisdom*.'" No one on the Harvard faculty of my student era could have been accused of that error.

Although I didn't realize it at the time, three values that became part of my work in ethics were being shaped. As a result of teaching a freshman writing course at Harvard for four years during my years in graduate school, I came to believe in clear, publicly accessible writing, not the kind typically found in philosophical or other disciplinary writings. Because of my work with Christopher Dawson, I could not thereafter separate debates about ethics from the background cultures in which they are historically embedded. Because of its glaring absence in the ethics curriculum at Harvard, I found it impossible to think about ethics without also looking at my own feelings, history, and psychological predilections. For my philosophical peers of the day, those concepts were exactly the sort of emotional clutter that should be removed from the mind to get down to the bare bones of reason.

Ethics as a subject matter invites self-deception, which must be combated, though doing so is not easy. Perhaps it's better to say that devising an ethic, personal or public, invites cultural captivity: being blinded or blinkered by the values of one's ethnic, religious, class, or ideological influences on public matters and all of those factors together with self-interest and egoism in one's private judgments. If losing my religious faith put me into the secular camp, having once had religion gave me the advantage of bringing to it a sympathy that many of my secular colleagues lack, which thins out and narrows their understanding of themselves and the human life about them. It gives me a nose for the lockstep secularists get themselves into, particularly if they entertain the delusion that they are more rational than the rest of us. The present crop of evangelical atheists—Sam Harris, Richard Dawkins, and the late Christopher Hitchens—provide as nice an example of smart people with little perception and understanding of the beliefs of others as one could ask for.

# 2

# My Own 1960s: A Decade of Transformation

In 1961 I left Harvard to take a job as an editor of *Commonweal*. Founded in 1924, the magazine occupies a unique niche in the American Catholic Church, known for its liberalism, its independence of the clergy, and as a voice of Catholic intellectuals. My writing had attracted the attention of the editors, and I was eager to accept their job offer, which I think I solicited. I arrived in New York with my Harvard dissertation still unfinished, saw my role as an editor only as a temporary stop on the way to teaching philosophy, and brought with me a strong Catholic faith.

But by 1969 I had received my Ph.D., lost my religious faith, and left *Commonweal*. I knew I wanted to be some kind of philosopher, but not in a university and not doing the kind of theoretical ethics, speaking mainly to other philosophers, that was the standard professional route. Although I could hardly foresee what would happen to me during next eight years at the magazine, I could also could not guess just how interesting they would be. Not long after I arrived at Commonweal, Pope John XXIII opened the Second Vatican Council in November 1962, and that Council continued until November 21, 1965. The Council stirred up great hopes for reform in a liberal direction and under the leadership of a lively and charismatic pope, John XXIII. For the editors of *Commonweal* it was a feast of news and articles, many of which I wrote.

But competitive with the Council for our attention was the war in Vietnam, which had escalated with a sharp troop increase in 1961. Although the magazine supported the war for a few years, by 1965 we had turned against the war. In the meantime, the first Catholic president, John F. Kennedy, had been assassinated in 1963. His candidacy in 1960 had notoriously stirred up a great deal of conservative Protestant opposition, which saw in Kennedy the opening wedge of papal power and a threat to the separation of church and state. Simultaneously, many in the Church—both in the Council and outside of it—were trying to break away from a long tradition of belief in a special role for it in society, one that had little use for the separation of church and state and that took upon itself the right to set forth moral rules for society, not just for Catholics.

The civil rights movement, escalating rapidly in the 1960s, and Lyndon Johnson's Great Society administration, responsible for Medicare and Medicaid in 1965, were fully in line with *Commonweal*'s liberal reputation and strongly supported by the magazine. More troubling was its ambivalent stance toward the authority of the church over individual conscience and church polity. That's where my particular story with the magazine begins.

## My First Book: On the Catholic Layman

While still at Harvard I had begun my first book, *The Mind of the Catholic Layman*, published in 1963 (my earlier book in 1961, *Christianity Divided*, was an edited collection of papers). I don't know where he heard of me, but Erik Langkaer, an editor at Scribner's (and editor also of Flannery O'Connor), approached me with the idea for the book. It was meant to be a history of laymen in the American church and a forum for my ideas about their role. I knew little about all that when I started the book in 1960, but I hired a research assistant, did much reading and the book was published in 1963.

What I learned was that despite high-minded declarations over the centuries about the importance of the laity, their reality was a lowly status—not just second-class citizens but hardly citizens at all. It was the duty of the laity to financially support the church and to send their children to parochial schools, but to leave all administration, finances, and especially all theology to the priests, bishops, and popes. Obedience to authority was an obligation that could not be evaded. Even if it is hard to determine exactly when the popes have ever used their power to speak infallibly (a power recognized by the First Vatican Council in 1870), that doctrine says much about the politics of the church and the way its authority has always been maximized—and always by the prelates and popes that would be its beneficiaries.

The politics can be seen in the right of cardinals to elect the pope, that same pope who has the only authority to appoint cardinals. The cardinals for their part have been chosen from among the bishops by the pope. It is a perfect model for running an authoritarian organization, religious or political. At the top is a pope who is called both "the servant of the servants" and the "holy father" at the same time. At the bottom are those servants, the laity, who are given no power whatsoever to break into the sacred hierarchical circle, skillfully organized to keep them out and successful for centuries in doing so.

### Upsetting the Theological Apple Cart: An Educated Laity

Although the laity had been educated to respect clerical and episcopal authority, two developments made that increasingly difficult. One of them was the simple reality that well-educated Catholics not only knew how to read but also how to read theology. "There has inevitably appeared," trenchant Church historian Monsignor John Tracy Ellis wrote in 1962, "a closer scrutiny of all that pertains to the Church, a sharper and more critical turn of mind which makes the educated Catholic layman . . . a quite different person from his unlettered immigrant grandparent of two or three generations ago." Eventually, but gradually, nothing would remain off-limits for that "critical turn of mind." The other development was the need for Catholics to find their place in American society, to discover ways to make their religion compatible with the separation of church and state, and perhaps even more important, to persuade their Protestant neighbors that they had the same freedom of conscience that all other Americans had. But if they wanted to make such a claim, they had to deal with a hierarchy and a Rome that looked upon such freedom as wrong and dangerous.

Efforts at the end of the nineteenth century by some priests and bishops to begin to confront that tension had mixed success. An extraordinary Catholic Lay Congress held in Baltimore in 1889 was, at least indirectly, meant to take on that challenge. One of the organizers, prominent convert and journalist Orestes Brownson, said that the congress provided the opportunity of "proclaiming to the world that the laity are not priest-ridden." Although the Congress did not in fact challenge any major church doctrines, it did arouse the suspicion of the bishops, who had to be convinced that such a Congress would not be dangerous.

Bishop John Ireland of St. Paul, Minnesota, took the lead in persuading a few other bishops and Cardinal Gibbons of Baltimore that such a Congress could, if properly supervised, be tolerated. That acceptance was facilitated by the creation of a committee of bishops to vet all of the papers to be delivered at the Congress. As one bishop put it, "Only the safest men should be selected to write, and they had better be left entirely free, after some preliminary advice." These conditions angered some of the lay organizers, but they gave way. Yet if the bishops were nervous that the laity would invade their theological turf, most of the presentations were of strongly liberal kind: the welfare of immigrants, the rights and needs of the working class, and the support of social justice. Traditional theological topics were not even approached. Even so, a papal letter to Cardinal Gibbons in 1899 sounded an alarm: some American values were beginning to infect the church, a threat that came to be known as Americanism, of which acceptance of the separation of church and state was a prime example.

### Liberal Political Policies and Conservative Social Values

The actual emphasis of the Lay Congress and the views of the bishops revealed a thread that has run through American Catholicism for well over a century since then: conservatism on matters of doctrine and personal morality and liberalism in politics and economics. That thread has remained stronger for the bishops than the laity, however. For the latter, dissent on moral matters has of late become more pronounced and political conservatism has been on the increase (and the once-solid support of Catholics for the Democrat party has been on the decline). An important way in which Catholics responded to the larger Protestant and secular culture has been, in effect, to accept many of its values, including that of a market culture. The hold of the bishops and pope on the laity has decreased and that of the condemned Americanism has increased.

All of these struggles were being played out in the church of the 1960s and among the *Commonweal* editorial staff. The older generation of that staff, publisher Edward Skillin and editor James O'Gara, were nervous about dissenting on doctrine and morality, though strong in their support of social justice and in their condemnation of the Vietnam War. The younger editors—an interesting and talented group that included a number who would move on to public notice in subsequent years (Peter Steinfels, Richard Gilman, Wilfrid Sheed, John Leo, and Michael Novak)—had fewer hesitations. Novak and Leo, as it turned out, later moved to the right politically—Novak to a position at the American Enterprise Institute and Leo as a columnist for the *U.S. News and World Report*, but we all shared a zeal in taking on what we believed to be the failings of the church. Moreover, by that time, even if the dissenting laity had little influence on the hierarchy, they were joined by a number of prominent American and European priests and theologians who became their allies, notably Hans Kung, Yves Congar, and Henri de Lubac in Europe and George Tavard and Charles Curran in the United States.

Along with *The Mind of the Catholic Layman*, I published two other books in the 1960s, *Honesty in the Church* (1965) and *The New Church* (1966), all written as I was finishing my doctoral dissertation. A collection of essays by a younger generation of Catholic intellectuals, *Generation of the Third Eye*, rounded out the decade. In 1965, our sixth child, David, was born, and my wife Sidney also published in that year her first book, taking on the church and feminism in *The Illusion of Eve: Modern Women's Search for Identity* and her first steps toward a Ph.D. in psychology. Our life was, as that list of activities will suggest, harried and hectic but invigorating as well.

We felt were taking on some of great issues of the day, and if we were in the solidly bourgeois wing of the 1960s—lots of children in a suburban town, Hastings-on-Hudson, New York, working ten hours a day, seven days a week—we were doing our bit as scholars and writers, not activists. We were not out on the streets but at our desks, now and then putting on parties for our friends, and endlessly changing children's diapers, but on the whole bookish types. On occasion I could lose my cool, notably when one of my children systematically cut up a number of chapters of the draft of my dissertation, requiring that I entirely write again some sixty pages or so. That was, I had to think, maybe his way of casting a vote about me as a father. (It's okay, John. I long ago forgave you.)

## Fomenting Dissent

In my various books, I wrote about some of the issues that were to preoccupy us, particularly those that were appearing in the church. My book
on honesty in the church did not focus on particular doctrinal matters
but rather on its institutional organization. The honesty in question was
twofold. One branch was the public failing of a self-protective church
intent on preserving its image of doctrinal consistency and rectitude, its
covering up of clerical and Episcopal misconduct, and its embrace of some
of the worst features of the surrounding society, notably its racism. When
my father was the manager of the radio station WWL in New Orleans,
owned by the Jesuits, he put a black preacher on for Sunday sermons.
Once the lay board of the station heard about that, he was ordered to
take it off the air. "Down here," they said, "niggers don't count."

Recall that most of the pedophilia cases uncovered in recent years
took place in the 1960s and 1970s, and along with their recent discovery
was that of the failure of many bishops to admit and face up to the
problem—instead, they often shifted the guilty priests out of sight to
some other diocese. Although it is not clear just how much Pope Benedict
XVI knew about the extent of the problem, at least one seemingly solid
report was that he hid an investigation of a priest in the name of "prudence." That was a common term often used by church authorities to
protect the laity from any suggestion of ecclesiastical scandal; knowledge
of it would be an "offense to pious ears." It was the hierarchy's term for
"coverup."

The other branch of the honesty issue I called that of private dishonesty, which I described in the following way: "The Catholic rarely knows
how free he is to express fully his thoughts, his doubts, his perplexities,
his hopes within the Church. He does not know the extent to which
those in authority will allow him to make known his inner life. Nor does
he even know how far the Church will allow him even to confront
himself." For those of us who thought of ourselves as Catholic intellectuals—a term that has all but disappeared in recent years—with a joint
obligation to the good of the church and to truth, we had a fundamental
conflict. Is truth to be defined as the church defines it, and is further
inquiry limited by its authority—or, as commonly understood in modern
societies, by that of following reason and knowledge wherever it takes

one? That has been part of America's secular and Protestant culture, and it is impossible for Catholics to not imbibe it as part of their lives in a pluralistic society.

The church's opposition to that culture for much of its early American history would come to seem stifling and anachronistic to later generations. In too many ways it was worse because it mirrored, albeit in a more benign form, the way in which fascism and communism had required the faith and obedience of their followers. Much of the debate between the young and the old in the *Commonweal* editorial offices centered on those questions of freedom and authority, and they also played out in the media by the debates at the Vatican Council. No longer could the church so easily get away with public dishonesty, and no longer could the Catholic laity live in good conscience with their private dishonesty.

### *Commonweal*: The Revolution that Failed

While those debates were rocking the church and the *Commonweal* editors, I tried to incite a change in the magazine's place among American journals of opinion. We should, I contended, be more ambitious, aiming to equal in prestige and influence *The Nation*, *Encounter*, *Commentary*, *Dissent*, and *The New Republic*. The Jewish magazine *Commentary* had managed, under the editorship of Norman Podhoretz, to do just that, which should be our aim also. I got a cool reception and generated considerable friction with Jim O'Gara, the editor.

He and the earlier generation of editors were comfortable at the top of the Catholic totem pole, and that was good enough for them. The term "laid back" might have been coined to describe their working style: 9:00 to 5:00 five days a week, nothing carried home for work at night or on weekends, no evenings of drink and talk with other journalists at the White Horse Inn in Greenwich Village, and no contact whatsoever with the leading intellectuals of the day clustered in Manhattan (save for Michael Harrington). The great struggles of the day about the left and anti-communism, the internecine wars among American liberals pitting Freudianism and Marxism against each other, and the outbreak of feminism were hardly more than the distant rumbling of cannon fire from battles they had no part in.

I got nowhere with my reform effort. Many years later, in an article describing the struggle with O'Gara, Wilfrid Sheed described the older editors as "Christian Gentlemen." As the ringleader of the revolt, I was described by Sheed as someone who did not share their leisurely pace. I had, he wrote, "no such cruising speed, but more a man of extremes, of large enthusiasms and exasperations that might, if acted upon, have given our whole enterprise a nervous breakdown." I have never thought of myself as a man of extremes, but agree that I am subject to fits of "large enthusiasms and exasperations."

## The Contraception Struggle

Both the staff debates at *Commonweal* and those within the church reached a peak with the use of contraceptives, culminating with two clear signals. One of them was the 1968 papal encyclical *Humana Vitae*, which decisively condemned the use of contraceptives. Pope Paul VI overruled a heavily lay commission he had appointed to study the problem, a majority of whom supported contraception. The other event was the widespread evidence not only that by that year a majority of the married laity were using contraceptives but also that they did so with considerable support from a large number of theologians, some bishops, and even cardinals and many priests as well.

Most ordinary parish priests neither supported the pope from the pulpit nor made any effort to challenge those parishioners using contraceptives. In 1964 the *Commonweal* published an entire issue on the problem and in 1965 it came out in favor of a change in the church's stand. I edited a book on the subject—*The Catholic Case for Contraceptives*—and Michael Novak edited a book of a similar set of essays by married couples, *The Experience of Marriage*. By the fall of 1964, participants in the Vatican Council were openly debating the issue. What brought about the change in the lay attitudes and among so many of the clergy? It provides an interesting example of the ways in which some long-standing moral values can change. Surely among the reasons was the fact that married couples who were otherwise faithful Catholics were finding it economically difficult to procreate children without limit—as good an example as any of the power of economics to change behavior and long true with demographic patterns—but no less difficult to live a celibate life in the near vicinity of a spouse. The separate beds of my parents' era, and the division of much informal social life into separate spheres of males and females, may have made it easier.

Seven children (one died) was our limit, and no one could claim that we had not done our share. No doubt important also was the acceptance of contraception by the rest of the American population. It was simply not considered a moral issue at all—just common sense. Many conservative Catholics have in recent years blamed most of the sexual promiscuity of the sexual revolution and the post-1960s years on contraception. But my parents made clear that contraception, even if not very effective, was common among Catholics in the 1920s, and priests blamed it for a low French birthrate in the 1880s. But demographers make a good case that economics is a decisive variable in family size. Much to my astonishment, many of my Yale classmates in the late 1940s—particularly those from wealthy families—were well into a kind of sexual freedom that many thought arrived only in the 1960s. Whether for economic or other reasons, my wife's parents urged us to end our procreative excess early in our marriage, along with our fellow married graduate students at Harvard, who basically thought we were crazy to have so many children.

The papal author of *Humana Vitae*, an unmarried male and a celibate, did not have strong experiential credentials to talk about marriage and procreation, and he was not helped by esoteric and unfamiliar natural law arguments. The pope and some traditional church teachings were on the losing side of a well-publicized struggle. It was not the first, nor surely the last, such occasion. The assault on the hierarchy's virtue and character occasioned by the more recent pedophilia revelations had earlier seen an assault on its credibility as a teacher of morality. As a long-time opponent of euthanasia and physician-assisted suicide, I cringed a bit when the Catholic bishops issued a statement against such acts in 2011. They were not ideal partners—perhaps as likely to scare off potential supporters as attract them.

## A Waning Faith

During the mid-1960s my Catholic faith began to slip, together with my theism. Many Catholics began drifting away in those days, and hundreds of priests left the church to get married or join another church. As I watched all of that happening, I realized that my experience was a little different. I simply lost interest in religion. I had plenty of complaints about the church, and loudly proclaimed them, but I liked Catholics as serious and good people and had many priests as friends (and still do). But I increasingly found that I could not pay attention in church—my mind was always wandering—and that theological talk of all kinds simply bored me. My mind and spirit were drifting away, much as my earlier enthusiasm for swimming and transportation economics had. That was a surprising turn for someone who had been called by a later church historian "perhaps the most influential laymen of the 1960s" (and a surprise to me to be so designated). By the end of the 1960s, that was all behind me.

Concurrently, I began to think that the whole Christian story made no sense. Why would a supposedly omnipotent and omniscient God create such strange, often evil and irrational human beings and then choose to send his son to be our savior, as if that was a good way to manage the problem of original sin and a fallen humanity? And why, for those who have been the victims of human evil, could it be possible to eventually wipe away all their tears in an after life? Could those who had watched their children being butchered or burned in genocide have *their* tears washed away, or the tears of their dying children? It was not a plausible story or an attractive one. The whole idea of a God came to seem implausible as well, and I ceased to believe it. But what is my answer to the question, "Why is there something rather than nothing?" I have no idea, and the explanation that it just happened ex nihilo is as implausible to me as to say God created it, and I have never heard of a plausible third option.

Yet I in no way share the anger or hostility that many atheists or agnostics feel toward religion. I believe that people are religious for three reasons, either alone or in combination. One reason is that they have, or once and unforgettably had, a powerful experience of awe or mystery, almost compelling them to believe there is more to life than the deliverances of ordinary experience. Abraham Maslow called that a "peak experience," and Freud spoke of an "oceanic" feeling. Another reason is that through religion, many achieve some greater insight into the meaning of life and comfort in living it that is unmatched by anything else. Still another reason is support of a congenial group of people who share a common way of life that is more important than whatever belief and doctrines may have given rise to it. In fact, they do not need to fully agree with the communal beliefs to find the group supportive and his or her presence in it acceptable. Just as many Jews have long described themselves as cultural but not religious Jews, it now seems possible to speak of cultural rather than doctrinal Catholics. How long either can endure in that state is uncertain in the face of pluralism, tepid religiosity, and interfaith marriage. All religions are having trouble keeping the young.

I have an analogy. It is well understood scientifically that homeopathy cannot have any medical efficacy at all. But for someone suffering from a chronic pain that modern medicine can do nothing about, and for whom homeopathy provides relief, it would seem irrational to give it up on the grounds of its scientific implausibility. Is it better to suffer than to employ a treatment that, according to reason, cannot work—but that does make a sick person feel better? The religious believer who is in a similar situation, in which all reason is against religion but all of his experience is for it, has good grounds to continue believing. The philosopher William James said something similar in *The Will to Believe.*

I can appreciate all of those reasons for belief and, although this is a large generalization with some exceptions, I find that I admire my friends who are religious believers more than the hard-core secularists I know. They seem to me kinder, more generous, more exploratory in their thinking and far less individualistic in their way of living with other people. Although I am not drawn to conservative religious believers, who I consider unlikely to practice self-examination and prone to closed minds in my experience, I long ago concluded that I would prefer to live in a society with liberal—essentially secular—values but in a neighborhood of religious conservatives. Believers in liberal values would be more likely to push for higher taxes if I and my kind were poor. The latter would reject the taxation but be more likely to take me in and buy me food. Religion for me seems in the end wrong but not irrational. Many bad things have been done in the name of religion, but even more in the name of science and reason—our secular deities—and of course many good things as well. But religion has no abominations on the efficiently organized scale of a Hitler or Stalin. Popes and inquisitors seem amateurish in comparison.

## Is Religion Necessary for Morality?

Clearly, even the most religious believers can (if they try) think of some unbelievers whom they admire, and there is enough substance in the history of secular thought and philosophy to put together a moral and worthy life. But even if that can be true of individuals, can it also be true of secular, nonreligious communities and societies? Yes, one can plausibly answer. We can see that perfectly well in many notoriously secular societies. The less religious countries, notably the Scandinavian ones and France, have a low church attendance and belief in God that is matched by equally low murder, theft, crime rates, poverty, divorce, and death rates. If they are on a slippery slope, they have not gone as far down as the United States, and not nearly as far as the most religious sections of our country.

Yet there is more than can be said. One line of thought is that secularized societies are living off the residual fat of religious cultures. The novelist C. P. Snow once said that "the scientist has the future in his bones." Perhaps it could be said also that the "secularist has the religious past in his bones." The late sociologist Philip Rieff contended that the real grip of culture lies in the "unwitting part," that which we display and embody but hardly note it happening. If that is the case, then ironically perhaps there is no way of knowing whether religion still has force, but is not directly visible, in the secular consciousness.

The main force of religion lies in the communities it creates, which—if tight and coherent enough—will shape and reinforce the ethical norms of that community. It was much easier to hold on to my religious values when I was well embedded in the Catholic community, where I did not hear about other ways of understanding the world. It was not the secularism of Yale (which was at best faint, despite what William F. Buckley, Jr. said) or that of the Harvard philosophy department (where it was strong) that shaped my thinking but the simple fact that there were competing views of the world and ethics, most having some plausibility. There was a Catholic community at Harvard, of which my wife and I were active participants. But it did not hold us in line nearly as well as some of the Irish-Catholic ghettos in Boston (South Boston and Dorchester, for instance) held their residents. The Mormons were a more tight-knit community at Harvard than the Catholics, and the Orthodox Jews even tighter still.

Yet if societies can flourish without religion as a foundation, those that have it as moral base have too often been compromised by their relationship with the state. Often the state can use it for its purposes even better than the church can for its ends. The dominance of the English church by Henry VIII or of the Spanish church by Franco are only two examples of the Faustian bargains required when religious power gets too close to secular power. It needs also to be said, however, that political regimes that seek to destroy religion do so out of a recognition that religious values can often effectively stand in moral judgment on dictatorships.

As the historian Richard Overy has shown in his book on the similarities and dissimilarities of Hitler and Stalin, *The Dictators*, they clearly shared two passions: that religion had to be destroyed and science put in its place. "Both systems," he wrote, "shared the conviction that moral norms are not universal or natural or the product of a divine revelation. The moral universe of both dictatorships was founded not upon absolute moral values but on relative values. . . . The only absolute reality the two systems acknowledged was nature itself." Religion was a potentially dangerous rival in rejecting such a belief. Yet even though the Catholic and Protestant churches offered some resistance to communism and fascism, and had some notable martyrs, they had been the beneficiaries of government sanction and largesse for too long prior to the arrival of those ideologies to be able to mount a strong resistance. That said, the evangelical atheists of our day who are virulently antireligion and enthusiastically pro-science should perhaps feel a little uneasy in having Hitler and Stalin as predecessors in that brotherhood. I doubt they will welcome that suggestion.

**The Insight of Tony Judt; The Failure of Left and Right**

I end this chapter with a most insightful comment by the late historian, secularist, and atheist Tony Judt in response to an interviewer, Christine Smallwood, in a 2010 piece in *The Nation* who said that she came from a religious background. She said that it seemed to her "that people on the left are so embarrassed by the language of morality that they've ceded the ground to the right." Judt responded by saying, "I totally agree. I think it's a catastrophe for both sides. What it means for the left is that it's got no ethical vocabulary. What it means for the right is that it smugly supposes it's got a monopoly on values. Both sides are completely wrong."

Judt then goes on to say that he came out of "a secular dissenting Jewish background" but with the "same thoughts of the old dissenting churches . . . in which there was a natural correspondence of social values and ethical criteria. And the divorce between them has been one of the disastrous results of the last half century." I would like to think that bioethics might help to bridge the gap Judt points to. We tried to introduce morality into medicine and biology when it appeared that science and positivism had pushed it aside.

By 1965 I had arranged to reduce my work load at *Commonweal* in order to do more of my own writing. I then took a six-month leave to teach at Brown University in the Department of Religious Studies. That was the beginning of the end of my interest in a teaching position as a career. New York had spoiled me, in great part because the editors and writers who made up my new professional community were livelier, more fun, and more venturesome than most of the academics I met at Brown. For the editors and writers I worked with in New York, the evening was just starting at 9:00 p.m. For the academics 9:00 p.m. was the time for everyone to go to bed. With my workload and many children, I was not actually able to hang out much with them, but even during the daylight hours they exhibited an energy and vitality I rarely encountered at Brown. Possibly my experience was unique and maybe I met the wrong people there, but I spent enough time as a graduate student and visitor to many universities to convince myself that they could in some circumstances be more an impediment to a serious intellectual life than a benefit. That conviction, as we will see later, had a significant bearing on my belief that the Hastings Center would be better off as an independent, free-standing center than part of a university.

### Taking On the Abortion Issue, and Learning Something about Advocates

From about 1965 through 1968, I was gradually pulling away from *Commonweal* and the church but was still caught up in the many religious struggles of the day. The next book I wanted to write brought about my final break with the magazine, not because of the topic of the book but because I had decided that having rejected teaching as a goal, I had also tired of editing. I had to find something else to do, and the book turned out to be a bridge to that unknown future.

The book was on abortion—*Abortion: Law, Choice, and Morality* (1970)—a topic that had grown in importance during the later 1960s as a number of states legalized it and that was of course a source of much controversy. As far as I could make out, no philosopher had taken it on; it was the province of theologians, lawyers, feminists, and doctors. Yet if I did not want to be an academic philosopher, neither did I want write a book aimed at them. I wanted it to be a serious book but one intended for a broad public, lay and professional.

Nor was it my instinct to start with the ethical arguments. I felt it necessary instead to immerse myself in the history of the issue, the way it was treated by the law around the world, and to understand what role it played in the life of women (feminist or not). One might call that an inductive approach, simply understanding it as a universal social phenomenon first of all and then determining how best to think about it ethically. That was to become the way I wrote all my books on ethics in the future. It was a break with the characteristic way those trained in moral philosophy usually worked, which was to steer clear of the messy underbrush of moral experience and to reduce the issue to the bare bones of arguments, propositions, and thought experiments. I had too much earlier exposure to literature, history, and the social sciences to find that a satisfying way to think about ethics.

I started writing the book leaning in an anti-abortion direction, but that approach gradually changed as my research proceeded. The change came about in great part because of what I learned in my research. A friend suggested that I should try to get a grant from the Ford Foundation, which had a program on reproductive health. I got the grant, which gave me the money to write the book. Hardly less important was their offer to give me virtually limitless travel money so that I could see for myself what was going on around the world. I took two trips, including a grueling three-week trip to Japan, India, Iran, Israel, Czechoslovakia, Sweden, and Denmark. On another trip I went to Mexico, Colombia, and Chile. I went to each of these countries because they had different cultures and different laws. One of my stops was in Prague, in August 1968, one month after the Soviet invasion. It was a gloomy place, filled with tanks and forlorn pictures of soon-to-be-deposed Prime Minister Alexander Dubcek in every store window.

What I discovered from my travels and my research was something of a surprise. No country liked the laws that it had, whatever they had. Japan and the Czech Republic, I learned, had unlimited legal abortion and a large number of repeat abortions (up to ten to twelve for many women). The medical experts in those countries said they were disturbed by the pervasiveness of the procedure, particularly by the medical damage of the repeat abortions (not at all in helped in Japan by the doctors who performed abortions working as a lobby to keep contraceptives illegal). In India and Latin American countries, where abortion was against the law, there was a high rate of illegal abortions with much medical damage as well. I could find no one who thought that was a good situation. The Scandinavian countries had a middle way, an "indications" policy that required women to get government permission for an abortion. The anti-abortion forces disliked it for its laxness and the pro-abortion proponents for its restrictions.

Something gradually dawned on me, however, regarding the situation in countries where it was illegal. Three features became clear. The most obvious one was that every such country had a high rate of illegal abortions, and that nowhere (save for Romania) were the laws enforced. In the United States, it took little searching to find doctors who would do abortions, with little fear of the law. My mother told me that had been common in the 1920s when she was growing up. Another feature was that most of the women seeking abortion did so because they already had more children than they could care for and they lacked knowledge of or access to contraceptives. Finally, a large number of women felt that the conventional male-female relationship, marked by female subservience, was one that makes it hard to say no to males. They had little choice about getting pregnant in those circumstances, with many men refusing to use condoms.

My research for the book took two years, and it came to 524 pages, some 300 of which were my research findings. The sections on ethics concluded that under some circumstances (not many), abortion could be morally justified but that under all circumstances the law should leave women free to make their own choice. I was persuaded to go in a pro-choice direction not by the usual women's rights arguments but, as it turned out, by my interpretation of the social context of women's lives. There was the tacit acceptance of abortion, represented by a universal failure to enforce laws against it, and the willingness of women to literally risk their lives with unsafe abortions—usually not for their sake but that of their existing children. My book was praised for its legal conclusion and was cited in a footnote in the 1973 *Roe v. Wade* Supreme Court decision.

### Abortion as a Moral Problem, Not Just "Personal Choice"

The pro-life forces of course rejected my arguments, but I had a problem with the feminist advocates of abortion. I wanted the law to make abortion legal, but I also contended that the abortion decision was a moral choice to be made with full seriousness and for good reasons. In that vein, I also said that in addition to leaving women free to make the choice, we needed to at least have a national discussion on what would count as a good or bad choice. I stepped well over the tolerance line with that proposal. Some feminists told me that because the choice was a "personal" one, there was no moral judgment to make. In response to that contention, I pointed out that part of ethics encompassed our personal lives, how we lived them, and the choices we made. I did not get far with that one. Other feminists conceded that, yes, there is a serious moral decision in principle that needed to be made, but said that in practice women were already too burdened with problems to have the time or energy to consider them. It was unfair and oppressive to even suggest—much less demand—that they wrestle with the problem. That argument was old-fashioned paternalism in the guise of women's freedom.

I had two other memorable run-ins with feminists. One of them was during a cocktail party. The women began discussing a prominent New York state prosecutor known for his public advocacy for legal abortion. He was also known behind the scenes as a person who had forced some of his romantic partners to have abortions. That story led to a general discussion of men they knew who had coerced women into abortions. I was surprised by the stories, saying that the public should know more about such things. But the political strategy, rigorously adhered to, was to say that it was chauvinistic men who were keeping women from reproductive freedom. So, I was told, "We will never say such things;

they would hurt our cause." I was evidently a naïve philosopher unaware of the higher truths of advocacy for good causes. The fact that public opinion polls showed that by a consistent majority, more women were opposed to abortion than men and that young males were the most in favor of it was not mentioned in the advocacy campaigns, either.

A later study by the Alan Guttmacher Institute in the 1980s found that some 40 percent of polled women said that they had been coerced into abortion (a study that was not repeated). My wife once observed that in our suburban community, mothers of pregnant young daughters were as like to coerce abortion as men. A number of demographic studies over the years have shown that husbands have tended to be more resistant to having children, or more children, than women.

Another memory was that of complaining about the euphemisms used to describe abortion, with "terminating pregnancy" and "emptying the uterine contents" being the most popular. I was met with outrage when I said that "killing fetuses" would be more accurate. I was met with no less indignation once when I asked a group of women (this was during the Vietnam War) whether they thought that the pilots of B-52 bombers, killing people from 35,000 feet, should be forced to see up close what they were doing—a popular antiwar contention. "Absolutely" and "of course," they responded! Did they then think it was a good idea for women to see pictures of what happens to a fetus during an abortion as part of trying to make a decision about having one? "Absolutely not— what an outrageous idea. How can you even make such a suggestion!" I was also enlightened once to be told that although I thought it was morally permissible to kill fetuses under some circumstances, only someone with a Catholic bias would give dozens of pages of a book over to agonizing about such a trivial issue as the moral status of the fetus. I quickly add here that I consider the single-minded elevation of abortion to the status almost of genocide by the Catholic bishops—while taking no responsibility for the violence and even murder that such rhetoric encourages—is not something the church should be proud of.

The phrase "a personal choice," common then and now among those on the pro-choice side, seemed to me to be a marker for a way of talking that deliberately empties the word "choice" of any moral content, entirely dependent upon what a woman wants, as if that is a moral principle in its own right and by definition a good choice. A 2011 article in the *New*

*York Times Magazine* discussed the decision of women who know they are carrying twins as a result of in vitro fertilization (IVF) to abort one of them. One of the women said, "If I had conceived those twins naturally, I wouldn't have reduced this pregnancy. Somehow making a decision about how many to carry seemed to me just another choice. The pregnancy was so consumerish to begin with and this became just another thing we could control."

## Wariness about Advocates

Perhaps unfairly, I came away from such encounters with a deep-seated wariness about having serious ethical discussions with people for whom advocacy in their own interests dominates their lives. They have made up their minds, they will tolerate no opposition, and they will quickly become angry when pressed about thoughts and ideas that stand in their way. In the early days of the Hastings Center, we developed an informal but helpful rule about inviting prominent advocates to our meetings, regardless of what side they were on: don't invite them, we know what they will say, and they are prominent because they are single-minded and adamant about their positions. Instead, invite someone with the same views, but who is not a leader, and someone with a willingness to talk openly about weaknesses in his or her position.

My pro-life wife and I, who occasionally agreed to public debates on abortion, made it a rule to specify the problems and shortcomings of our own convictions in our presentations. In such a debate at the Harvard Medical School, many in the audience were surprised that we would do such a thing, more or less unheard of in abortion debates. For my part, I was surprised when many listeners—male and female doctors, medical students, and interns—said that our debate was the first time they had ever listened to an "intelligent" (much repeated) otherwise obviously liberal woman present a pro-life position. I wondered where they had been for the past decades.

## What I Think I Learned from Examining Abortion

What did I learn about ethics from the abortion wars? First, my perspective on abortion was shaped in great part by my examination of the kinds of familial and male pressures that left many women, if not most, feeling that they were trapped and helpless, with abortion seemingly their only way out. Yet I don't think I recognized that so much at the time as I did later in trying to explain to myself why I had changed—why I went one way with the arguments rather than another.

Second, my wife and I disagreed on the issue and argued about it almost daily for three years. As a pro-life feminist, she is opposed to war, capital punishment, the oppression of women, and supportive of gay marriage. Her view is that women, knowing historically how women have been treated as chattel by powerful males, should not use their power to rid themselves of unwanted fetuses as property to be disposed of. It is a comparable misuse of power. She also noted once, a bit wryly, that feminists were arguing that women were tough, resilient, ready for any challenge—other than an unwanted pregnancy. I couldn't really disagree agree with her views, which seemed to me sensible and plausible. But I saw the problem of women and abortion from a different and overriding angle.

We also noted that, fully aware of all the arguments, data, and convictions on both sides, we nonetheless disagreed, and that was not easy to explain. She was religious, but none of her pro-life reasons were. Together we published a book, *Abortion: Understanding Differences*, a collection of papers by women from both sides that tried to get at the reasons why they differed rather than where they stood on the law or the moral status of the fetus. My wife had organized the conference leading to the paper and, not accidentally, I was the only male present.

Third, although philosophers and theologians have developed nuanced, careful arguments about abortion that are useful in the class room and valuable for those who take the trouble to read them, when the issue becomes public and enters the courts, two changes occur. One of them is that passion, anger, and single-minded advocacy usually emerge. Civilized dialog soon gets overwhelmed. The other is that underlying ideologies come to the fore, shaping the way people frame the issue, the kinds of arguments they are likely to accept, and their attitudes toward those on the other side. Abortion is an uncommon type of ethical dilemma, as close to a black-or-white choice as can be imagined. The law can establish a range of legal options, but a woman contemplating abortion can either want it or reject it. There is no comprising third way.

Moreover, abortion elicits particularly strong passions because it is seen as part of a larger moral drama. For pro-choice women, it is often taken to be the litmus test of women's right to control their own lives and bodies. For pro-life advocates, it is a test of how we value human life and dignity, particularly that of the most helpless among us. It is extraordinarily difficult to resolve that fundamental kind of clash. That's why it has ethically remained uncommonly intractable. Although public opinion polls have recently been slightly more pro-life than earlier, they have remained remarkably similar over the years, showing a population divided, and the pro and con arguments of today are not much different than those of forty years ago. After about fifteen years or so, Sidney and I became worn out by the abortion battles (public and marital), declared a truce, and mutually resigned from the whole debate. That was a great relief.

I might note, however, that in 2010 my wife Sidney was invited to a large conference on abortion at Princeton that brought together pro-life and pro-choice groups. I was not invited, and that hurt a bit. My 1970 book was called at the time the best book ever written on the topic (well, at least two reviewers said that) and sections of it were regularly reprinted for years. I consoled myself by recollecting that I had once said in response to well-meaning, faintly critical comments on my large number of children, that I would wager that "my children would have a longer shelf life than my books." I was right.

### The Population Council: Reducing Birth Rates

In 1969, just as I was finishing the abortion book and beginning work to found the Hastings Center, I was offered a one-year job at the Population Council in New York. Heavily supported by the Ford Foundation and the Rockefeller Foundation, it was the world's leading private organization for family planning policies and contraceptive research. Its work was primarily focused on developing countries, and one of its missions was to find ways to reduce the medically and economically harsh impact of large families—six to eight children per woman, with many of them dying in infancy, was not good. But trying to change that pattern raised some serious ethical issues. The president of the Population Council, well-respected social scientist Bernard Berelson, asked me to think about those issues and to give them some policy advice. I was hardly an expert on the ethics of family planning and population policies, but no one else was, either. My favorite kind of issue has always been one that is brand new, lacking in any previous literature, and waiting to be made sense of—and this was one of them.

What had become evident at the Population Council before I had arrived was that earlier policies had failed to make much difference. The most prominent ones were those rooted in a technological fix, most notably that a policy of providing a bit of education and many contraceptives. That strategy—"parachuting condoms"—was derided by many skeptics in the population-limitation ranks. It did not change long-established ways of life in agricultural cultures for whom large families were a necessity. But if those ways of life were deadly for mothers and children, with high death rates for both, would it be morally legitimate to in some way legally coerce people to have fewer children? China, as was well known, had had an excessively coercive one-child family policy. Their solution ran afoul of the reigning principles of the family planning movement: the right to make one's own choice about how many children to have. It would thus be a violation of basic right as enunciated in UN documents.

How about searching for some acceptably fine line between education and manipulation? A common strategy with women altogether ignorant of family planning methods was to use the pretext of house-to-house health surveys as a way of deliberately insinuating possibilities that they had never heard or thought of: "How do you control the number of children you have?" "What are you talking about, there is no way of doing that?" "Do you know what a contraceptive is?" "No, what is that?" "It is a way to have sex without having children; would you like to learn more?" That was an effective strategy. Because it was reasonable to assume that most poor women with six or seven children would have preferred to stop having more, it did not seem to me to be wrong, even though the method of getting in the door to talk required some contrived ways of starting a conversation. In any event, the general failure of family planning programs led to a later shift at important UN conferences to an emphasis on women's education, which correlates most directly with family size. That change in policy meant that the earlier ethical dilemmas of trying directly to influence procreation for the most part disappeared, and birth rates fell. Only in sub-Saharan countries do they remain high.

I close this chapter by noting that I had a hard time getting the researchers at the Population Council to take seriously any talk about ethics (though Bernard Berelson was an important exception). They were essentially data collectors and technically oriented policy analysts and were almost visibly uncomfortable talking about anything to do with the language of ethics. It was not that they rejected my talking about ethics, but they were so far outside of that kind of discourse that they usually listened to me with at best puzzled expressions on their faces. That was all the response I could get. Nothing I said interested or aroused them. It was soon obvious to me why the earlier fixation on contraception availability had been a failure: a technological fixation utterly innocent of cultural and value-related issues. But I did get an article on ethics and population limitation published in *Science* magazine, the most eminent science journal, and I think that may have impressed them. That does not mean they read it.

# 3

## Giving Birth to a Center: 1969–1979

I began thinking about a research center on ethics in 1967. At first the idea was to have a general focus on ethical issues of all kinds, but that came to seem too broad. As time went on, my work on abortion and at the Population Council, as well as a number of conferences in the 1960s—many organized by scientists on the likely impact the genetic developments and the new technologies that were changing medicine, often called the "new biology"—led me to narrow my focus to ethics and the life sciences. Many of those conferences concluded by saying "someone needs to be thinking about the challenges in an organized way."

At a Christmas party in 1968, I cornered a friend and neighbor in Hastings-on-Hudson, the psychiatrist Willard Gaylin. I told him about my idea of a research center focused on medicine and biology and asked him if he would help organize it. Always the enthusiast, he thought about it overnight and called the next day to say he would. That was the beginning of a forty-five-year partnership and friendship, with no serious disagreements during all those years. Although neither of us had any experience in starting much less managing an institution, or raising money for one, we had a serene confidence that we could do it. If we could not, that would be our fault: the issues were there, they were gaining public and professional attention, they demanded concerted attention, and they were inherently interesting. How could we miss? Even so, I can recall the anxiety expressed by a few friends, mainly academics, who said that with six children at age 39 I was too old to take that kind of gamble and should look for a tenured teaching position. Others, however, mainly Manhattan publishers and writers, where tenure is unknown, said that "I was a young guy and should go for it."

## Our Log Cabin Days

I call that first year our log cabin era, set in a well-to-do suburb. Was it hard, many have asked? Yes, in the sense that we had to find money every year and were living on the edge, but no because our issues kept growing in importance and could not be evaded. We did not think we could possibly fail; our self-confidence, our chutzpah, sustained us. At one critical moment my mother lent me $2500, and for the first year the center was in my house—in our bedroom, to be exact—with additional files and machines in Will's house.

In 1971 we moved to an office building in Hastings, just upstairs from the quarters of a popular dentist and internist. Will and I agreed that he would be a part-time president and I would be the full-time director and manage the day-to-day work of the Center. We wanted a somewhat fuzzy division of labor to deal with an immediate problem: just what kind of expertise did the leadership have? What credibility did a philosopher have to work on medical issues? How many patients had I ever treated? I was frequently asked. But my colleague is a physician, I would answer. And what credibility did a physician have to speak about ethics? He could point to me. Together we had both medicine and ethics, which got us past that hurdle.

Four early decisions had to be made. The first was our name, and we chose the Institute of Society, Ethics and the Life Sciences—somewhat of a mouthful. Early on, we had to cope with widely different notions of what ethics is all about, and many thought it had to do with only individual behavior. We added the word "society" to counteract that view. After a few years, we informally came to call ourselves the Hastings Center, in great part because we were too often called the "ethnics" institute and our field that of the "light sciences," and even the staff could not be reliably counted upon to know where the commas in our title went. The second was how to characterize our way of thinking, and there was immediate agreement the Center had to be interdisciplinary. The ethical issues quickly spill out beyond the discipline of ethics into law, medical and biological sciences, sociology and anthropology, history, and culture. No one field could claim ownership.

## The University Dilemma

The third question was whether we should be part of a university. Most thought it self evident that only a university would be right. Where else could we find talent and the necessary library resources to do our work? But a few warned us against universities as political and bureaucratic as well as inhospitable to interdisciplinary research. We took little convincing of the latter view, encouraged by a similar attitude on the part of one of our first supporters, John D. Rockefeller III. We were quickly assured of the correctness of our choice by the failure of two university efforts at the same time, those of Yale and Penn, to get a bioethics program started. We had been warned by some foundations that we could never compete with their efforts and prestige. As it turned out, they lost, bogged down in committee meetings and outgunned by two fast-moving entrepreneurs who had to consult only a bureaucracy of themselves. We never regretted that decision. It would be many years before those universities had programs in bioethics.

The fourth question was: who should be our audience? Will and I had begun our writing careers in the 1960s with the trade press, aiming in both our cases for an audience of academics and the reading public for our books. Will's writings covered a wide range of subjects, including a study of the Vietnam War resisters who chose to go to jail and bias on the part of judges. Our bioethical issues seemed ideal for that mix, combining a complex array of moral problems and dilemmas that touched on difficult technical questions and no less on ordinary lives. Not soon after we opened our office, I got a call from the health officer of a county in California. That county, he said, had limited funds for the illness of children, but he had two children who needed organ transplants to save their lives. The cost of those transplants would wipe out his entire children's budget, leaving nothing for any other child. What should he do? I was staggered by a question that seemed unanswerable at the time and cannot now recall how I responded—no doubt with something vacuous. But it was evident that a question of that kind needed robust discussion and debate and that our audience had to encompass a wide public and professional audience—a goal that fit well with our interdisciplinary commitment. Good work of that kind needs plain English to cross disciplinary lines.

## Ethics: Resistance, Suspicion, and Skepticism

We had from the start the support of some eminent scientists and physicians (Franz Ingelfinger, Ernst Mayr, René Dubos, Theodosius Dobzhansky), many of whom we recruited simply by calling them out of the blue and asking for a chance to talk with them. We also encountered a fair degree of suspicion and skepticism among many of their colleagues. The suspicion was that as outsiders we would invade the temple of medicine and conduct witch hunts to root our wrongdoing. Part of the skepticism stemmed from the belief that if medicine had some ethical problems, these would best be handled within the profession.

As one distinguished professor of medicine put it in 1968 when Senator Walter Mondale was attempting to establish a presidential study commission on the emerging ethical issues, he saw no need to gain the help of "theologians, philosophers and others to give some direction . . . I cannot see how they could help . . . the fellow who holds the apple can peel it best." Senator Mondale was startled by that kind of reaction. "All we are proposing is a measly little study commission to look at some profound issues. . . . I sense an almost psychopathic objection to the public process, a fear that if the public gets involved, it is going to be anti-scientific, hostile and unsupportive." Only in 1973 did Senator Ted Kennedy, following up on Mondale's effort, succeed in establishing the National Commission for the Protection of Human Subjects of Biomedical and Behavioral Research. The revelation in 1972 of a medical research project at Tuskegee Institute in which approximately 600 black syphilis patients were for 40 or more years deliberately denied efficacious treatment even when penicillin eventually became available was an important reason for the work of the commission.

Yet there was another kind of resistance to ethics in our early days: skepticism about its solidity as a discipline. That resistance was harder to combat and has continued to lurk below to a much lesser degree below the surface for many decades since then. Many physicians, educated in the 1940s and 1950s—in the era of positivism and A.J. Ayer's *Language,*

*Truth, and Logic*—believed that ethics was nothing more than an expression of emotion, that truth lies in scientific facts and ethics in the trackless wasteland of subjectivity. For others, ethics was thought to be religion, either openly or in disguise, and for still others a mischievous (but double-edged) sword with which to uncover political or economic malfeasance—in the other political party.

Even those who agreed that the ethical dilemmas of medicine and biology were real had trouble believing that the discipline of ethics was up to resolving them. Many foundations we solicited bluntly expressed that view. As they perceived it, ethics has no clear methodology, is little more than a collection of competing and usually irreconcilable theories, and has not in 2,500 years managed to come to some definitive agreement on right and wrong, good and bad, virtue and vice—that is, on just about everything about ethics. There is some basis for all of those perceptions, and part of the story of the development of the field was the need to show that progress could be made and that plausible ethical policies can be fashioned. Could bioethics tell the California doctor how to allocate his scarce resources if the same problem arose today? Not easily, but it could help him work his way through it in some orderly way.

If our interest in ethics was what made our institution unique, the widespread ambivalence about ethics was a burden. And if ethics itself was a puzzle to many, bioethics as a field was unknown. The word "bioethics" did not come into common usage until the early 1970s, coined by a scientist not even in the field: Van Rensselaer Potter in his book *Bioethics: Bridge to the Future*, well after the topics that gave it that name came before the public eye. I was not drawn to the term, mainly because I wanted (as did some others) to be called a moral philosopher, not a bioethicist. Ironically, however, the Library of Congress officially added "Bioethics" as a subject—citing me as the authority for doing so.

Even so, not a single foundation, and barely any government agencies, had programs anywhere near our interests. That meant we had to talk our way in, making a case that if they weren't interested, they should be. Our most effective approach was not to talk about ethics directly, but to pose two questions to the foundation officers, most of whom were at least middle-aged: "Do you have elderly parents and, if so, have you worried about their old age and end of life care and what to do for them?" Most said yes. And, "Do you have adult children worried about having children because of infertility or anxiety about the health of their prospective children?" Most said yes, and we said that those are the kinds of issues we worry about as well. They got the point and often helped us, even when we were obviously outside of their announced interests.

**Our First Grants, by Way of Some Wayward Children**

Our first grant was for $15,000 from the National Endowment for the Humanities, the one place that was open to research in ethics. The grant, however, was a matching grant: we had to find another $15,000. But luck counts in this world if one knows how to make the best of it. One day a Hastings neighbor called to complain that my children were running through his yard and would I please ask them to stop doing so. I had no doubt the complaint was valid, apologized to him, and to change the subject, asked who he was and what kind of work he did. "I am John Maier, Director of the Biomedical Division of the Rockefeller Foundation," he answered. "Well, isn't that interesting," I enthusiastically said. "Let me tell you what I do."

Not only did that exchange lead to the matching grant from the Foundation, but we were also encouraged by that success to understand that excitement and conviction opens doors. Our next piece of luck came shortly thereafter. Two of our early supporters, Alfred and Blair Sadler, twin brothers then at the National Institutes of Health (and authors of the government act that put individual's wishes for organ donations on their driver's licenses), told us they had a classmate from Amherst, David Lelewer, who had just joined the staff of John D. Rockefeller III and whose job it was to give Rockefeller philanthropic ideas. We were one of his first ideas, and Rockefeller's $30,000 was our first gift. Shortly thereafter, Elizabeth Dollard, a prominent lawyer friend of Will Gaylin and a benefactor of the Yale Law School, made another large contribution.

In later years, my younger colleagues at the Center persistently complained about the need to get grants, a tiresome and boring part of the Center's work. Will and I didn't feel that way. We liked coming up with project ideas, enjoyed trying to sell them to often skeptical foundation officers and potential donors, and as it turned out, rarely failed if we got a chance to be heard. We were, as entrepreneurs, admittedly not the equals of Bill Gates and Steve Jobs, who were getting started around the same time, but we did almost as well in our own way. Or maybe it could be said that they did almost as well as we did.

There have been a number of arguments over the years about the origin of bioethics, and a memoir is a time-honored (if not necessarily reliable) way to set the record straight. One approach to the history is to single out the issues as the starting point, and for many the 1960 dialysis episode and its life and death selection panel is a good place to start. For others it was Henry K. Beecher's mid-1960s revelations about nefarious medical experiments or the 1972 Tuskegee story. Along with Beecher, legal scholar Jay Katz at Yale and philosopher Hans Jonas wrote about human subject research in the late 1960s, and Princeton theologian Paul Ramsey published a probing study entitled *The Patient as Person* in 1970.

## Creating an Institution, Legitimating a Field

If it takes the appearance of issues, scholars to write about them, and public interest in them to constitute the beginning of a field of inquiry, it also takes the creation of institutions to make that field an organized whole. That is exactly what the Hastings Center did in 1969, adopting as its agenda the ethical problems as they presented themselves and encompassing all the disciplines of pertinence in an organized, systematic fashion to deal with them. The Kennedy Center Institute of Ethics at Georgetown University came along to do much the same thing in 1971 (with a more academic bent), running a spectacular event at the Kennedy Center to announce its birth, and featuring everyone from Mother Teresa to Beverly Sills and many Nobel laureates added for good measure. I was assigned Alice Roosevelt Longworth, Teddy Roosevelt's witty and notorious daughter, as my dinner partner before the main event. "No," I told her when asked if my children had ponies as she had at the White House, "no ponies."

At one point, we courted the Kennedy family to support us. At a meeting with Ted Kennedy, Sargent Shriver, and Eunice Kennedy, we were asked if we did deep, slow, and serious work. Absolutely, I replied. Well, what if the senator asked you for some fast, even overnight, work: could you do that? Easily, I said. We did not get a penny. I was later told that our fatal error was that we did not offer to put the Kennedy name on anything. I don't credit us with some lofty integrity for that omission. Babes in the woods that we were, it never occurred to us. And Georgetown's Kennedy Center already got there first. Around the same time, some universities invited us to join them. We were flattered by their attention, but the small print of the offers stipulated that we would have to find our own space, bring our own money, and put ourselves under their administrative rule. That was not an attractive offer, and it took little character to reject it.

With some money in hand, our first organizational need was to put together a staff, and we did that by hiring Robert M. Veatch, who was just finishing his Ph.D. work in medical ethics at Harvard, and Marc Lappé, a biologist with a degree from the University of Pennsylvania (whose wife, Frances Moore Lappé, had just written her much celebrated book, *Diet for a Small Planet*). Our original idea was that we would put together a national group of experts to be called our Fellows and that our research work would be organized by the staff and carried out by the Fellows. As there was no field at the time, we sought the Fellows by word of mouth, looking for those who had written on the issues (not many) or those we thought might be attracted to them.

Princeton theologian Paul Ramsey was an obvious choice; he in turn suggested that we ask Leon R. Kass, a young physician at the NIH with an additional degree in biology, to work with us. Kass had created something of a stir by attacking in the *Washington Post* a scientific proposal for research on human cloning. Henry K. Beecher, whose revelations about wrongful human experimentation had attracted much attention, was another obvious choice, as was René Dubos, an interesting Rockefeller University biology professor whose book *The Mirage of Health*—arguing that illness, decline, and death are intrinsic to human life—had a profound effect on my own thinking in the face of utopian scientific scenarios promising to rid us of those evils. Alexander M. Capron, a recent graduate of Yale Law School and a protégé of Jay Katz there; Renée Fox, a sociologist of medicine at the University of Pennsylvania; Paul Freund, of Harvard Law School; geneticist Kurt

Hirschhorn, at the Mt. Sinai School of Medicine; biologist Robert M. Morison at Cornell; Nobel laureate James D. Watson; and Theodosius Dobzhansky, a geneticist from the Rockefeller University were just a few of the people we invited to serve as Fellows or board members. Even if they did not know us personally, they liked the idea of what we were doing.

**A Helpful Social Style: Drinks, Families, and Dancing**

That we were without great difficulty able to put together a first-rate group of supporters served as a counterpoint to the skepticism about ethics noted previously. Along the way Will and I devised, almost intuitively, a social style that was a great help. We held many of the early meetings in our houses, told the participants to bring their spouses and children, and took everyone to a local Irish pub that featured dancing after the meetings. Our aim was to distinguish the Hastings Center from the conventional professional societies that all of them belonged to but also, by working to create friendly personal relationships, to defuse the tension and controversy that often marked our heated topics. Well-organized drinking, eating, and carousing the night before our behavior control meetings on psychosurgery to tame violent behavior—pitting buccaneering neurosurgeons against psychiatrists—did much to soften everyone for the next day of serious talk, an instance of our homely form of behavior modification. There was one important historical outcome of those meetings. The psychosurgeons complained that it was unfair for psychiatrists to criticize them for failing to do long-term studies of patient outcomes because psychiatrists did no such studies either. They were right. That charge led one of our Hastings participants, Gerald Klerman, to lobby the federal National Institute for Mental Health for outcome studies, an important development there.

A memorable moment at one of the meetings was when the prominent neuroscientist José Delgado from Yale described his experience in coming through U.S. customs on a return trip from Spain. He went to that country, he said, because it was easier there to get hold of intact heads than in the United States. "What do you have in those bags," the custom officer asked. "Heads," he answered. The officer then checked a book of acceptable items and could not find the word "heads." "Here," Delgado said, starting to open a bag, "let me show you." Sounding horrified at the prospect, the officer said, "Never mind, go on through."

## Choosing Our Initial Topics

Although we expected our staff members to write their own books and articles, their main duty was to organize and direct interdisciplinary group projects. We chose for our initial focus four broad areas of research, each of which, we judged, would be of fundamental importance and of long-standing interest: population and reproductive biology, behavior control, end-of-life care, and genetics.

They turned out to be good choices. At the time, the great population concern was that of excessively high birthrates in developing countries but with a parallel focus on American birthrates, stimulated by Paul Ehrlich and the Zero Population Growth (ZPG) movement. We did early work with the United Nations Fund for Population Activities (UNFPA), the first international project for the Center. We also discovered how hard it was to talk about the ethics of population control in that context—that is, in an institution fragmented along cultural lines, riven by political fights, and with a heavy bureaucracy fostered by those struggles. We admired the tenaciousness of the staff members for putting up with all that. We saw firsthand how hard it is to work through ethically difficult problems in a highly charged political context.

The advent of prenatal diagnosis in the 1960s and research on in vitro fertilization in the early 1970s brought great public and professional attention to reproductive biology. In the developed countries, population had declined with the end of the baby boom era in the mid-1960s. With that decline came smaller families, rising health, psychological, new economic demands in the raising of children, heightened talk about genetic engineering of babies, and pre- and postpartum screening of babies. A sense of nervousness and anxiety about having and raising children appeared in the 1970s, far greater than what my wife and I and most other couples had when we started in the mid-1950s: the medical development brought new expectations, heightened health anxieties, and the emergence of procreative choices unimagined earlier.

By "behavior control" we meant a variety of scientific efforts to manipulate human behavior, and particularly to reduce violent behavior.

Crude forms of psychosurgery—an ice pick inserted through an eye socket into the brain, for instance—had been introduced with no ethical oversight or control at St. Elizabeth's mental hospital in Washington, as had a variety of behavioristic strategies building on the work of B. F. Skinner. A Hastings neighbor, prominent African American psychologist Kenneth Clark, was calling for a drug to control violence. That desire led to some provocative discussions about the place of aggressiveness in human life and whether in fact it would be a good idea to attempt to eliminate it. Many commentators, while agreeing that it would in some sense be good to eliminate violence, countered that some aggressiveness is necessary for human life, at the least for self-defense. But no one could calculate just how much, and the idea of an antiviolence drug went the way of many utopian speculations—just fading away.

Genetics found an obvious place among our research areas because of the rapid expansion of scientific and public interest in the wake of the discovery of the double helix structure of the DNA molecule by Watson and Crick in 1953 and the advent of recombinant DNA and gene splicing in the 1970s. But the dream of genetic manipulation and the use of genetic information for clinical purposes had been in the air long before that. Greater control over the genetic influence on health, the enhancement of desirable human traits, and the elimination of those that are deleterious were all part of an excitement about genetics that saw it as the most likely way to achieve the dreams of human improvement and even the mastery of human evolution, and they were laid out on the research and media platter as irresistible delectables.

They were also accompanied by darker shadows and worries—too much power, too much hubris, too much recklessness—giving rise to a ubiquitous anxiety phrased as the danger of "playing God." That term made little sense, even to theologians, but the eugenics movement of the late nineteenth and early twentieth centuries, later taken up by Adolf Hitler, underlined the potential dangers. That kind of worry was not shared by the researchers or their financial backers. Most in fact knew that much of the utopian talk, even if some came from scientists, was for the foreseeable future mainly hot air. Yet the advent of predictive and personalized medicine in recent years, aiming to diagnose and treat the sick based upon their unique genetic makeup, has been called the newest and most exciting frontier of medical progress.

## Two Early and Eventually Divergent Bioethics Streams

If those were our main research areas at the outset, it is possible to distinguish two streams of bioethical interests that soon became apparent. One of them was traceable to the series of conferences organized by scientists in the 1960s, placing the emphasis on the potential of medical and biological progress to change our view of human nature and the way we live our lives. Those were the issues that had stimulated my interest. The parallel development focused on more immediate policy and clinical challenges, encompassing human subject research, the doctor-patient relationship, prenatal diagnosis dilemmas, and end-of-life care.

The latter set of issues soon came to overcome the former and drew the greatest foundation and media interest. It soon became evident to us that it would be easier to find money for policy matters than philosophical reflections on the future of human nature. Nonetheless, the shadow of nuclear weapons, still strong in the aftermath of Hiroshima and Nagasaki, made it possible to see scientific progress and technological prowess as capable of evil as well as good. It was far easier in that era to raise questions about progress than it was by the 1990s, when anxiety or pessimism about technological progress was more quickly dismissed as Ludditism.

In addition to establishing research groups in the four noted areas, we initiated an effort to bring the teaching of ethics to medical schools. At the time, only the Roman Catholic schools had such courses, though a few secular ones were beginning to show interest. The Columbia University College of Physicians and Surgeons, where Will Gaylin was a clinical professor, let us start a course there. It didn't last long. Some medical students reported how disappointed they were that there was no kidney dialysis unit at Columbia-Presbyterian Hospital, which Gaylin and I had not been aware of, and about which we had no opinion at all. But it interested the students, so we talked about it. Word of that classroom discussion got back to the dean, who accused us of stirring up trouble and hurting the school's reputation. We were told to cancel the course. The same dean was later enraged at Gaylin for an article he wrote on cloning for the *New York Times Magazine*. Although it was hardly favorable to cloning, the dean felt that it sensationalized the topic and posed a threat to the school's ability to get research grants. It was our first clue about the growing and often deleterious dependency of medical schools on research grants, the results of which include a significant downplaying of teaching, which brings in no money, the way research grants do.

Undeterred, we organized a national conference on the teaching of medical ethics in 1972, which was as far as we knew the first such event. There was some persistent opposition to actual courses in ethics, often taking the form of faculty claims that ethics was taught in all the courses (which medical students told us they had not noticed) or that ethics in medicine was based on the role modeling of senior physicians, not something that warranted a course.

Our main advice to those organizing courses was to steer well away from semiretired, distinguished faculty members, who were usually addicted to anecdotal clinical war stories. One pleasant memory was an encounter with a scornful professor of internal medicine. Ethics, he said, was a waste of time: it never gives a straight answer to anything. I then asked him how he would handle a question by a medical student about how to treat high blood pressure. He said it would all depend on the age of the patient, other medical conditions, and likely counter-indications to the available drugs for treatment. In other words, I said, you wouldn't give the student a straight answer but would instead give him a range of questions to ask and things to think about—and that's just what those of us in ethics do with individual cases. He said, "Okay, you got me." By the early 1980s, our effort and those of others had paid off and most medical schools had some kind of program or course. It was a special treat in 2011 to help initiate a program under the auspices of the Yale-Hastings Program in Ethics and Health Policy in medical ethics at the Yale University School of Medicine, the last major medical school in the country to do so.

## On a Fast Track: The Emergence of Bioethics in the 1970s

As with the rise of courses in medical ethics in medical schools and a parallel development at the undergraduate level, the 1970s saw a rapid number of other developments in the field. The efforts of Senator Mondale culminated in the establishment of the National Commission for the Protection of Human Subjects of Biomedical and Behavioral Research

(1974–1978). It was precipitated in part not only by the efforts of Senator Mondale but also by a controversial recommendation by an NIH study panel that newly delivered live fetuses be used for research before they died. Senator Ted Kennedy, Chairman of the Senate Labor and Welfare Committee, held hearings on a bill introduced by Senator Jacob Javits, the ranking Republican member of the committee to require the NIH to establish review committees on human subject research and to provide grants to medical schools to improve the teaching of medical ethics. I testified at one of the hearings and said, "We simply cannot afford as a species to stumble about blindly in a thicket which may produce more thorns than flowers." That was hardly a profound comment, but it was emblematic of the pervasiveness of an anxiety—not just mine—that scientific progress, and particularly its messianic features, were as much to be feared as to be embraced.

That was not my only encounter with Senators Kennedy and Javits. In 1973, I became interested in a problem, now familiar, that was only then emerging: the control of health care costs. With a grant from the newly established Robert Wood Johnson Foundation, we established a research project on that issue, bringing together a number of young economists who would later become important figures in health care, notably Alain Enthoven, Victor Fuchs, and Thomas C. Schelling.

In 1975 Will Gaylin and I met with Senators Kennedy and Javits to discuss the bill they had introduced into the Senate for universal health care. The ethical basis of the bill was a "right to health care." Senator Kennedy said, however, that they had a problem openly espousing such a right. "We have," he said, "no way of talking about how to set some limits on that right." I said that we had not heard that problem even discussed, to which the senator responded, "No, we can't talk about that, it's too hot to handle." He then said that difficulty was something the Hastings Center should take up. It was a flattering suggestion, that our staff of five persons should take on an issue that could not be discussed in the U.S. Senate. Their reform bill did not make it out of committee, and it would be ten years before I returned to cost control. It is still hard to talk about rationing and limits in Washington, even when everyone agrees at some high level of generalities that it is necessary.

As it happened, health care reform was not part of the initial burst of national interest in bioethics. But the 1970s was a time of great excitement in medicine, bioethics, and the nascent life of the Center. Organ transplantation (particularly of the heart and kidneys), in vitro fertilization, advances in prenatal diagnosis, the acceptance in law of a brain definition of death, medical progress and the accompanying moral dilemmas in saving low birthweight babies, and *Roe v. Wade* were only a few examples of a broad spectrum of emerging issues. I want to center my attention here on a few such issues that began to shape my ethical thinking, my style in writing about them, and on the development of bioethics: the Karen Ann Quinlan case, turning on the cessation of treatment of a comatose young woman; the recombinant DNA drama, bearing on a revolutionary development in genetics; and the entry into bioethics of philosophers, displacing theologians as the leading theoretical analysts of ethical problems.

## The Karen Ann Quinlan Case: The Legal Debut of Bioethics

In April 1975, Karen Ann Quinlan was brought unconscious to the emergency room of a New Jersey hospital. The 21-year-old woman was in a deep coma triggered by a combination of alcohol, barbiturates, and Valium. She was eventually put on a respirator and, after some weeks, was diagnosed as being in a persistent vegetative state with no likelihood of improvement. Her parents requested that she be taken off the ventilator and allowed to die. Her physician denied their request and the case made its way finally to the New Jersey Supreme Court. In March 1976, the Court decided that the ventilator could be turned off.

The case was important for the Center. Every one of the major actors in the case turned to us for advice, the hospital on one side and the family on the other side, and New Jersey state authorities in between. My splendid and prolific colleague Robert M. Veatch, the staff member responsible for our Death and Dying research group, came to play a central role, but all of us became involved in one way or another. The case drew enormous media attention and was historically important as the first instance in which a court upheld the right of a dying patient (or one for whom further life-saving efforts were judged to be futile) or, in this case, the right of a family member to terminate treatment. Taken off the respirator, Quinlan managed to survive for a decade, much to the surprise of everyone, not dying until June 1985. At the time, her condition, a persistent vegetative state (PVS), was hardly discussed, and traditional Roman Catholic theology regarded the cessation of nutrition and hydration as acceptable as turning off a respirator. But in Quinlan's case, that was not done; nor did her Catholic parents ask for it. Many decades later, the Church unwisely turned against such a resolution, much to the surprise and consternation of many theologians.

## End-of-Life Care: The Long Road Ahead

Our Death and Dying research group came to have a special importance for me, one that transcended the difficult legal and ethical dilemmas of terminating treatment. The first project of that group considered the definition of death, supporting the move from the traditional heart-lung cessation to whole brain death, but in the process learned how difficult it is to determine when someone has irrevocably died. To say that a person is dead for legal purposes when their brain is dead solved the legal problem in an acceptable way, but not the deeper problem of biological death, the shift from life to death, and from living to dying.

That last distinction—determining when a person had crossed the line between living and dying—would in coming years be critical with the care of critically ill, possibly dying, patients. The hospice movement, initiated by work in the United Kingdom of the physician Cicely Saunders in the 1960s, came to the United States in the early 1970s, first put into place at the Yale–New Haven Hospital. Complaints about the dreadful care often given dying patients, particularly a failure to relieve pain, gave rise to a strong movement to reform that care. Three remedies were widely agreed upon: greater patient or surrogate choice in the termination of treatment, better training of physicians to treat the dying, and the development of hospice services and improved palliative care.

Yet as time went on, it became evident, at least to me, that the continuing failure of those reforms reflected not only a deep-seated resistance by patients, families, and physicians to acknowledge the coming of death but also the power of technological medicine to blur the line between living and dying. Such a medicine is very good at prolonging the process of dying with technological interventions that can almost always add a few hours, days, or weeks, to a dying patient's life. As one medical anthropologist, Barbara Koenig, discovered, for many doctors a patient is dying when there are no further interventions possible to save him or her. Death, that is, is a function of the failure of technology, not something that happens to the body. As German philosopher Hans-George Gadamer nicely put it, "The prolongation of life finally becomes a prolongation of death and a fading away of the experience of the self."

In that respect, I was beginning to be uncomfortable with the general trend in the care of the dying. The emphasis was almost exclusively on the right to choose at the end of life along with various other moves to improve care. Those moves were surely important, but sorely lacking was a public discussion to help people understand the place of death in life and thus what substantive content to give to their choice. Just when should I be willing to have treatment terminated, say, and what difference should it make if my loved ones resist that choice out of a desire to keep me with me? Hardly less lacking was a direct confrontation of medicine's de facto warfare against death, most prominent in biomedical research (but with a clinical spillover), and a key foundational premise of medical progress. I will develop that line of thought in chapter 5, but it was during this period that I started wondering just what the appropriate goals are for medicine and health care, particularly the place and priority of the struggle against death.

## Genetics: The Utopian Frontier

If end-of-life care was a clinical focal point, genetics was seen as a key to utopian medicine of the future. The early 1970s saw the emergence of a number of conferences on genetics and the formation of our research group on that subject. In 1971 I was asked by the Fogarty Center of the NIH to organize a conference on the ethical issues of genetics. Among the topics covered were prenatal genetic screening, gene therapy, cloning, and the potential for stigmatization that screening could bring. That was the start of a number of such conferences and an intensified debate about genetic possibilities and threats.

Most memorable was the controversy on recombinant DNA, popularly called *gene-splicing*, meaning the capacity to splice foreign DNA into the genome. It was a technique that promised great research benefits as well as possible clinical applications. It was also a source of ethical concern among many scientists because of the unpredictable nature of the results, primarily new forms of dangerous viruses. Two conferences at a California conference center organized by genetic researchers in 1973 and 1974 and called Asilomar, addressed those concerns. Together with a few members of our genetics research group I was invited to the second one, called Asilomar II. I felt too busy at the time to accept the invitation and have regretted it ever since. It turned out to be an historic event, in part because the research scientists themselves took the risk of bringing their worries out into the open, calling for a brief moratorium on the research. As a policy outcome, its recommendations were the foundation of a federal committee organized shortly thereafter to oversee the research.

Around the same time, my colleague Marc Lappé submitted a proposal to the NIH to support a Hastings Center project on it. We received an insulting letter from the director of the NIH Institute for General Medical Sciences. He said that our project idea was nothing more than "blue-sky" speculation by philosophers about a nonissue. We did not get the grant, but we did get an unsolicited letter of apology a year later saying he had been wrong. That was almost as satisfying as the grant we did not get. He was by then overwhelmed by the public debate, most notably in Cambridge, where Harvard's plan to open a recombinant DNA laboratory incited considerable community opposition. The mayor of Cambridge said that "they may come up with a disease that can't be cured—even a monster. Is this the answer to Dr. Frankenstein's dream?"

But there was an important fallout from the effort of the scientists to take on the ethical problem: finding the right balance between valuable research and public safety. A small group of prominent scientists, among them James D. Watson, said in the aftermath that it had been a serious error for scientists to make their worries public. Doing so had served only to incite the public to needless anxiety and was an obstacle to research. In later writings I characterized Watson's stance as an embrace of the "gambler's principle"—stop the ethical hand-wringing and get on with the research—over against the "precautionary principle," which in effect holds that scientists should look before they leap. Whether because of that backlash or other reasons, no group of scientists has since that time voiced serious reservations about any biomedical research. Nor has that happened much with bioethicists who, by the end of the millennium, were more prone to defend scientists against criticism than to push them ethically. Speaking truth to power ceased to have the force of the 1960s and 1970s behind it.

## The Philosophers Arrive, Displacing the Theologians

The advent of philosophers taking up bioethics was of special importance to me as a philosopher. Up through the late 1960s, bioethics (then still called medical ethics) was in the hands of theologians. That was not because of any religious invasion of the field but simply because the major religious groups—Protestants, Catholics, and Jews—had long traditions of ethical inquiry into medicine. Protestant theologians James M. Gustafson and Paul Ramsey, Catholic ethicists Richard McCormick and John Ford, and Jewish rabbis David Bleich and Moses Tendler all had a leading place in the emergent bioethical debates.

Prior to my entry into the field, there was hardly more than a handful of philosophers in the 1960s, which notably included my Harvard classmate Dan Clouser from the Pennsylvania State Medical School; Samuel Gorovitz, who became a dean at Syracuse University; and Hans Jonas, a German philosopher at the New School for Social Research in New York who had studied under Edmund Husserl and Martin Heidegger and was a friend of Hannah Arendt. In 1970, the journal *Philosophy and Public Affairs* was initiated by a group of young philosophers—among them Derek Parfit, Thomas Nagel, and Thomas Scanlon—aiming to bring philosophy more directly into public policy and to move beyond the emphasis on metaethics and linguistic analysis that had been the mark of Anglo-American analytical philosophy.

But the most striking and influential event was a six-week summer institute at Haverford College in 1974 specifically aimed at bringing philosophers into the field and organized by Samuel Gorovitz. It drew many of the major philosophers of the era, most notably Robert Nozick and Bernard Williams, and many younger ones who were to make their mark later. Almost all of them had been trained in the same dominant Anglo-American analytic tradition as I had but were now drawn to the ethical issues of medicine and biology, offering a wide range of new, important, and philosophically interesting problems. Unlike the editors of *Philosophy and Public Affairs*, whose intended audience seemed to be other academics, many of the philosophers at the Haverford institute wanted to be on the firing line of ethics, working directly with physician, researchers, and policymakers. Many of them came later to serve as the staff members of the federal presidential commissions on bioethics who began to be appointed after the mid-1970s.

## The Impact of the Philosophers

The coming of the philosophers to the still nascent field had, from my perspective, two decisive impacts. One of them was to quickly overshadow, and eventually to simply push aside, the moral theologians. They did so by means of different language and concepts, sharply contrasting styles of argumentation, and (with some exceptions) a strikingly secular outlook and open hostility to religious ideas. One of my great problems as director of the Center in subsequent years was to deal with that hostility in putting together our research groups. In many cases, I simply had to override their objections to including theologians, who had as much of interest to say as the philosophers. The other impact was to introduce the cool, impersonal, and putatively "rigorous" mode of moral philosophy. For our physicians (and for me) in the early years, Hans Jonas was the model of the wise philosopher. But his European training, his interest in Gnosticism, and his panoramic studies of ethics and technology did not impress the analytically trained. He had little standing in their eyes—and that judgment reduced their standing in my eyes.

The influence of the philosophers was soon felt. The National Commission for the Protection of Human Subjects was mandated by Congress to "identify the ethical principles which should underlie the conduct of biomedical and behavioral research with human subjects." Historically, the history of moral philosophy, going back particularly to Immanuel Kant in the eighteenth century, was that of framing rules and principles for conduct. Moreover, in the context of American public policy and government regulations, that was a congenial approach. In the case of human subject research, the 1947 Nuremberg Code developed by the prosecutors on the International War Crimes Trial was the historical precedent. Out of the deliberations of the National Commission came the *Belmont Report*, on which work began in 1976 and was completed in 1978, and which was then used as the foundation of federal guidelines. Its immediate aim was to set forth ethical principles for human subject research, but its findings were subsequently taken up for use more widely as principles for general bioethical application.

## The *Belmont Report* and the Four Ethical Principles

The original *Belmont Report* specified three principles—respect for persons, beneficence, and justice—with the final version put into shape by Tom Beauchamp of Georgetown University. Expanding on that list to encompass the additional principle of nonmaleficence (do no harm), Beauchamp and a colleague, James Childress, published in 1979 the first full-scale textbook on bioethics, the *Principles of Biomedical Ethics*, at the core of which were the four principles. Moral rules, they argued, are meant to deal with particular situations, with those rules in turn justified by broader moral principles, and those finally grounded in ethical theory. Noteworthy was the belief, which I accepted at the time, that bioethics should be grounded in moral philosophy and its way of going at ethical problems. This approach put to one side once and for all a competing view, advocated notably by the physician Edmund Pellegrino, that the ethics of medicine should be fashioned from the values, practices, and traditions of medicine, not from philosophical theory.

Although I initially supported the idea of a structure of bioethics fashioned on different levels of moral philosophy, I was from the first left uneasy by the four principles—all the more so when they seemed to be used almost obsessively and indiscriminately to solve ethical problems. Our journal, the *Hastings Center Report,* was for years flooded by manuscripts on all kinds of issues that made an almost mechanical use of one or more of the principles to solve all ethical problems, far from the nuanced use of them by Beauchamp and Childress. Later critics came along to take to task what came to be called *principlism* for a variety of shortcomings, most notably failing to have a way of setting priorities among the principles that would deal with conflict among them, such as between the interests of individuals and the demand of justice. Though sometimes derided as the "Georgetown mantra," principlism has had a long life, in great part because Beauchamp and Childress in subsequent editions of their book refined their approach and sought to deal with the critics.

But my uneasiness did not stem from the effort to define principles for use in decision making, but for two other reasons. One of them was that the four principles in the end could all too easily be reduced to one—respect for persons—usually understood to be personal autonomy—my right to make my own choices and fashion my own vision of life—a most congenial American value. The aim of justice seemed in the end to have as its health care goal that individuals received the care needed to exercise their autonomy as citizens. I came to see them as closer to political than ethical principles, that is, how we should treat our fellow citizens in our public life. They tended to block from consideration the substantive questions about those principles that a full ethical treatment required.

We ought to be free to make autonomous choices on important life issues, but just how ought we to exercise that freedom when we have it? What counts as a good or bad choice? That last question, as you may recall from my earlier abortion discussion, is exactly what got me in trouble with the feminists. People should receive equitable health care, but there is a prior question: what kind and quality of care should be available for fair distribution? Beneficence requires a judgment about what is *really* good for people, a question that pushes deeper than principlism is ready to go.

## Does Bioethics Require an Underlying Ethical Theory?

Still more troubling was the status of ethical theory, taken to be the cornerstone of ethical analysis and judgment. The concept of moral theory is itself ambiguous, open to a variety of meanings—for some a "guiding framework" (John Rawls) and for others the logical analysis of ordinary moral language or the discovery of "a valid of a set of valid moral principles." The most common view has been the invocation of two fundamental ways of organizing broad and contrasting views of morality: utilitarianism and deontology.

Utilitarianism in one standard version understands morality to be the search for the greatest good of the greatest number and that of maximizing pleasure over pain. Deontology focuses morality on the notion of our duty to follow moral rules as our highest ethical obligation. There have been many objections to both theories but they pose in one common understanding a basic conflict between an ethic of consequences and an ethic of moral rules, many of which rule out a consideration of consequences.

We may, that is, decide that some situations require us to lie to someone because of the possible harmful consequences for that person of telling the truth. When my mother was dying of cancer, the possibility of which had terrorized her for most of her life because of her mother's horrible death from the disease, we decided not to tell her the truth; doing so would, we judged, serve no useful purpose. A strict duty-based ethic would hold that we should have told the truth regardless of the consequences. But it does not take a very active ethical imagination to see the drawbacks in both theories or why, in practice, there seem some situations that demand taking consequences into account and others that seem to demand we do our duty, however unpleasant.

In short, not only are there many contending versions of moral theory, but each and every one of them has its critics and drawbacks. No decisive way of judging those differences or settling on a winner has emerged. That did not stop efforts by bioethicists in the early years to ground the field in some kind of theory, either in the traditions of medicine or, more decisively, in the ethical theories of moral philosophy. Many philosophers held that there could be no good bioethics that did not have a theory at its core. That search proved to be as elusive for bioethics as for moral philosophy in general. Nor was that the end of the theory difficulties. Even having a theory in hand did not necessarily offer any effective way to make the move to actual clinical or policy practice.

Tom Beauchamp in later years noted the decline of interest in moral theory because of all those difficulties and concluded on an ambivalent note. On the one hand, he wrote, "thousands of publications later, the grand promise of ethical theory for bioethics remains mainly promise." But then, on the other hand, he seemed to endorse a continued effort to find a theory, and particularly to find a way to connect that theory to practice, "a problem of greater urgency today than it was thirty years ago." He did not say why. My own experience in working with many

ethical issues, dilemmas, and decisions has been that the available theories are rarely helpful, being too large and general in scope to offer much
illumination with complex many-layered problems. They do not help us
establish the moral status of the fetus, the balancing of risks and benefits
in prenatal genetic screening, the meaning and scope of the concept of
human dignity, or the fairest way of organizing health care systems in
the face of ideological struggles.

## Try as I Might, I Could Not Take the Theory Debate with Due Seriousness

I relate that history of the theory debate in bioethics because, as it developed in the 1970s, I realized that I had little interest in it—it seemed
beside the point too often, of use neither in framing the question for
complex problems nor in offering a way to find a solution. Perhaps that
was because I was by then more than a decade removed from my graduate student days, when I had been required to take the theory debates in
moral philosophy seriously. More likely it was because I could never
make out the connection even then between theory and actual conduct.
It seemed like an abstract set of arguments and preoccupations that was
not grounded in the experiences of ordinary life, or even interested in
it—a kind of high-level "game" (as one of my Harvard professors put it)
for those who were, as with an interest in chess, drawn to such puzzles.
Just as it was not necessary to be a good person to do good ethics, it
was not necessary to have an ethical sensibility for what was in the end
a matter of good arguments and a skill in deconstructing the words and
concepts of morality—but independent of their social and cultural
context. I often felt of many philosophers, even some in bioethics, that
they were like musicians who were steeped in musical theory but could
not carry a tune.

As I look back on my 1970 book on abortion, I realize now what I
was not conscious of at the time: that I made no use of moral theories
at all, nor did I, in my style of writing, want to sound like a detached,
rationalistic analytical philosopher. The only explanation I can offer for
those omissions was that the theory debates I had learned about in my
philosophy classes had made little impression on me, offered little illumination for actual ethical problems.

One reason I moved away from the literary and argumentative style of academic philosophy is that I had become comfortable writing for a general educated audience as a *Commonweal* editor and had come to think that was the only audience worth writing for—and that doing so should appeal to academics as well. Only later, as mentioned earlier, did I become aware that was the way that Harvard philosophers in the late nineteenth century and the early twentieth century saw their audience. They did not write for other philosophers, and I did not want to do so, either. Moreover, I came to think that most of us, even professionals in ethics, think of our own moral life in ordinary language, not in the jargon of our trade. Louis Menand, writing about William James, caught my views perfectly when he wrote that James "never let go of the conviction that a philosophy confined exclusively to the academy is a philosophy not worth pursuing. . . . Some philosophers philosophize to philosophize, others philosophize to live."

### Ethics from the Bottom Up: An Inductive Approach

I also came to find it better to proceed inductively, so to speak—that is, working up from the concrete details of medical or societal problems to the larger ethical perspectives—rather than deductively from theories and principles down. What I came to appreciate—in the face of efforts by analytic philosophers to strip complicated problems down to the bare bones of well-formulated propositions suitable for technical analysis— was the importance of social, psychological, and cultural understanding of what the full scope of an ethical problem is. That stripping process can be called *reductionistic*, a notion I picked up from many scientists of that day who complained of reductionism in biology, moving away from the organism as a whole to its various parts, as if that strategy would reveal some hidden secrets and the solution to a biological puzzle. Until the failure of the human genome project in the 1990s to find a genetic basis for all disease and thus a royal road to clinical cures, reductionism was in the saddle. It may still be, but perhaps more sobered by that failure. I am not sure whether the philosophers (of a certain kind) have learned such a lesson.

My almost spontaneous suspicion of principlism came in the end to its embrace of individualism—not specifically to the concept of respect for persons, which seemed right, but for reducing that concept in its use to autonomy and for enthronement of choice as central to ethics as a whole, not just to end-of-life care and human subject research. Autonomy was to loom large as the reigning moral value, something more than a principle, in the bioethics taking shape in the 1970s. A book by Episcopal theologian Joseph Fletcher, *Morals and Medicine*, published in 1954, though quickly bypassed as the field of bioethics unfolded, caught in an oddly prophetic way some dominant themes of the emerging bioethics of the 1970s. "Choice and responsibility," he wrote, "are the very heart of ethics and the sine qua non of a man's moral status." The advances of medicine entail "control over health, life and death," a control that "is the basis of freedom and responsibility, of moral action, of truly human behavior."

## Yes, There Is Much Agreement, at a Certain Level, on Moral Truth

As I look back, I think I intuitively came to believe that we already possess in our culture and traditions some universal conceptions of right and wrong, of doing good and avoiding harm, which is also reflected in international instruments. That insight was developed by philosophers Bernard Gert and Sissela Bok. In lieu of some generally accepted ethical theory, probably never to be realized, our level of consensus on ethical virtues, rules, principles, and prohibitions gives us all the agreement we need to make good progress with most of the ethical issues of bioethics— and just about everything else as well. They rarely give us a reassuring certitude, but enough insight to act in a responsible, even if often contentious way. I particularly came to dislike "thought experiments"—the invention of "what if" and other types of imaginary scenarios.

Physicians, I discovered, could not stand such scenarios. They have real, and messy, dilemmas, and the elegant play of philosophers with thought experiments seems to them an evasion of the need to look ethical problems in the eye, often punching us in the face and demanding that we accept them in all their confusion and rational disarray. Three books I read in the 1960s and 1970s were influential in my suspicion of individualism and the combination of choice and control that were its marks, none of them philosophical. They were *The Mirage of Health*, by biologist René Dubos, contending that illness and death are an inherent feature of human life, open to limited control only; sociologist Philip Rieff's book *The Triumph of the Therapeutic*, which took the ethos of psychotherapy, making no moral judgments but aiming only at individual well-being, to be destructive of a culture of necessary restraint and limits; and historian Christopher Lasch's book, *The True and Only Heaven: Progress and Its Critics*, which deftly and somewhat pessimistically takes apart the value of progress, as important and preeminent a value for modern medicine as for many other features of a technology-dominated culture.

Over the first decade of the Center's life, two overarching questions had emerged for me. If death cannot be eliminated, if moral dilemmas cannot be solved by some bottom-line recourse to psychotherapy and individual choice, and if the control over our life that the idea of progress fosters is a god that can fail, then how are we better to understand our lives and the pursuit of health that is part of it? And if large-scale general moral theories and thought experiments are of limited help, then what might be more helpful?

Although I have cited three books as influential in my thinking about ethics, I should mention that I gained as much or more listening to people talk and to how they talked at our many conferences. We averaged about a conference every two weeks or so during that decade on just about every topic in bioethics and brought in talented representatives of every field and discipline. I helped organize most of the conferences and sat through all of them. As often as not, my notes were about other topics and ideas that the discussion stimulated in my mind, often having nothing to do with what I was ostensibly listening to.

Apart from my abortion book, published in 1970 but written in 1968–1969, I wrote only one other book in the 1970s: *The Tyranny of Survival* (1973). I had decided that, as often as possible, I would try to find topics that were new, hiding below the surface and waiting to be expressed and developed. The *Tyranny* book, which got hardly any notice at all, was just such an effort. Its aim was to contrast the cultural celebration of freedom of choice, strongly evident in the family planning movement and the culture of the 1970s, with that of an entirely different stream of thought visible in the population control literature. That latter stream, fed by the work of Garrett Hardin and Paul Ehrlich, pressed the contention that coercion and a denial of choice would be necessary to control dangerous population growth—a threat to long-run human survival itself. The tyranny of individualism pitted freedom of choice against the tyranny of survival needs. As it turned out, as mentioned earlier, that tension took care of itself in the population policy fraternity with the insight that the education and freedom of women would do more to reduce population growth than formal family planning programs. It remained to be seen how many other moral values and freedom of choice policies could indirectly achieve social and communal benefits. The 1980s would help me find that out.

# 4

# Coping with Success: 1980–1986

By the end of the 1970s, the Hastings Center had become well established, as had the field of bioethics. After a few years, we moved from our original office on Warburton Avenue to a building on the Burke estate owned by the Hastings-on-Hudson school district. That estate had been owned in the 1920s and 1930s by Broadway impresario Flo Ziegfeld and his wife Billy Burke, an actress famous for her role as Glinda, the good witch in *The Wizard of Oz*. I felt sure she would have approved of our work, though sometimes we felt most like the wizard, pulling levers behind a screen and talking in a way that projected a wisdom about large moral puzzles we did not yet have. *Time* magazine did a nice story about us that spoke of "dramatically handsome Willard Gaylin and elfin Daniel Callahan." Some years later, a friend of mine at the Kennedy School at Harvard, Mark Moore, said that he was tired of being called "cute" and aspired to look awesome. My wife said, looking at both of us, "I'm sorry, but short guys with curly hair will never look awesome." Nor dramatically handsome, apparently.

Our new building not only offered more space for a steadily growing staff but was also only few hundred yards from the local middle and high schools. That propinquity meant that our children could easily visit and work for us. Our interest in ethics did not go so far as prohibiting nepotism or paying underage kids less than a living wage. We were as well within walking distance of our homes, and my wife Sidney, who had, along with Will's wife, Betty, gone out of her way to feed and entertain a steady stream of visitors and conference participants.

Sidney gradually got drawn into our issues, writing on them and being invited to conferences. She was a commentator on a much-discussed 1971, somewhat inflammatory film entitled "Who Should Survive," which recounted the story of a couple who refused a simple operation to relieve a digestive obstruction in their Down Syndrome child that was necessary to save the child's life. The child was then allowed to die. The film was a composite of three cases at the Johns Hopkins Medical School, at a time when such children were still called "Mongols."

## A Marital Struggle and a Broken Promise

But Sidney had no aspirations to become a bioethicist. She aimed to get a Ph.D. in psychology and had already begun taking courses toward that end at the City University of New York (working with, among others, Stanley Milgram). We had agreed, when first married, that I would get my degree and, once established in my work, would stand aside to let her get her degree. Now that time had come, and I failed to keep my promise. I could see no possible way to relieve my workload at the Center, getting busier by the month and chronically, as in many a classic "soft money" venture, always forced to raise money. Even now, looking back, I cannot imagine how I might have kept my promise, but ethically speaking, that is not always an exculpatory excuse. Maybe I could have if I had tried harder.

So we struggled, argued, and managed maritally to muddle through. She received her degree in 1980, a wonderful accomplishment for her and 100 demerits for a husband who smugly prided himself on liking smart, ambitious women, who changed diapers in an era when men did not do that, and who had been proud of her for publishing a book on feminism in 1965, *The Illusion of Eve: Modern Women's Search for Identity*, and editing a collection of essays, *The Working Mother* (1972). Her own essay in that collection was written under a pseudonym—a charitable gesture to save me from disgrace. As women know, that kind of male weakness is an old story.

As the Center grew in size and influence, our need for money grew with it. By the early 1980s, federal grants were increasingly available from the National Endowment for the Humanities, the National Science Foundation, and the National Institutes of Health. A wide range of private foundations, none of which had programs in bioethics, helped us as well. The great and surprising exceptions were the many foundations that specialized in medical research and health policy. After an initial grant in the 1970s for work on ethics and health care, and in the late 1980s for end-of-life care, we got nowhere thereafter with the Robert Wood Johnson Foundation, the largest of these foundations. A staff member there told us it was mainly board opposition, not staff opposition, as they worried that our issues were too controversial. An officer at the Howard Hughes Institute said much the same thing, only more colorfully: "If we give money to you, we might get picketed. It's much safer to support improved high school science teaching." I had to admire him for his willingness to say something so patently wimpy.

With the other major medical foundations, we never got in the door far enough to be turned down. Their staff members were mainly health care economists and policy analysts who seemed to have little use for ethical reflection. But we did well with private donors in our annual fundraising campaign and, in the mid-1980s, Edwin C. Whitehead, the founder of a medical device company called Technicon, gave us $1 million for a capital campaign that managed to gain another $1 million. He designated most of his estate for the creation of the Whitehead Institute in Cambridge, now a major biomedical research center. He could be an unpleasant man, and he was no intellectual. After he complained once too often about the *Hastings Center Report*—"I can't read any of that crap"—I asked him to resign from our Board of Directors. He did, and I have wondered to this day how I got myself to do that. It would be nearly twenty-five years before we found other contributors in the same league.

## The Golden Year: 1981

The year 1981 stands out in memory as one of the high points in the history of the Hastings Center. We had on staff a number of young scholars who would go on to be leaders in the field—Arthur L. Caplan, Ruth Macklin, Ronald Bayer, Bruce Jennings, and Thomas Murray—and distinguished visiting scholars included Stephen Toulmin from Oxford, prominent for his writings on ethical theory; Gregory Vlastos, a renowned Plato scholar from Princeton; Jeanne Guillemin, who went on to become well known for her work on biological warfare and terrorism; and Gerald Dworkin, a leading philosopher from the University of Illinois–Chicago.

What we did not have on the staff or among our visitors were social scientists. Renée Fox, a distinguished medical sociologist at the University of Pennsylvania, was one of our first board members, and she nagged us to find more social scientists. But the relationship between philosophers and social scientists was sometimes strained. Many years later, when I was teaching in Division of Medical Ethics at the Harvard Medical School, part of the Department of Social Medicine (led by Arthur Kleinman), it was hard to not notice the hostility of the social scientists there against bioethics, particularly the philosophers. The failure of most philosophers to pay attention to the social and cultural features of the ethical life was taken to be a basic flaw in their way of thinking. I was a bit more tolerated than most. I shared their distaste for analytic philosophy and usually worked a fair amount of social commentary into my writing.

By the early 1980s, physicians and lawyers were increasingly coming into the field, drawn by its importance for their disciplines and along the way diluting the earlier sway of philosophers. They were disinclined to worry much about the ethical theories that captivated philosophers. By the end of the millennium, in fact, the flow of philosophers into the field seemed to have declined and philosophy had returned to its old narrow and ingrown ways, becoming in the process one of the easy targets for university budget cutting.

## The Eastern and Central European Opening

Meanwhile, inquiries were arriving from philosophers and physicians who wanted to come to the Center from Central and Eastern Europe. They were interested in bioethics but had no courses in medical or other schools, could not afford books or journals, and had received no education on our issues. Could we help them? We did so by gaining a grant from the George Soros Foundation. Soros, a multibillionaire, was a Hungarian by birth and, little known by the public, a philosopher in his earlier, pre-investment career. We organized workshops in Prague, Pecs (Hungary), and Dubrovnik; initiated a visiting scholar program; and sent over books and articles. It was a great pleasure to receive an honorary degree for that work in 2008 from the Charles University in Prague.

But all that was before the Velvet Revolution, and there was a back story. Although the interest in bioethics was real, there was a parallel, underground agenda: to discuss medical ethics was to allow a way of talking about otherwise taboo topics, that is, freedom and justice. Communism had introduced corruption into the health care system, especially bribery of physicians to get good care and reserving the best hospitals for party members. During that same era, we held a number of workshops in Europe on bioethics.

### Human Subject Research: The First Bioethics Service Industry

Back at home in the United States, human subject research protection, picking up after the work of the National Commission, became one of the most active areas of bioethical activity, a small industry in its own right. Every organization carrying out biomedical or behavioral research must have an institutional review board (IRB) to make decisions on the ethical acceptability of research protocols. There have always been struggles to make IRBs work well despite being heavily dependent on unpaid volunteers, often inadequate administrative support, and excessive workloads. Questions about the meaning of informed consent from research subjects and risk-benefit calculations have never gone away, and the consent forms for subjects have become increasingly long and borderline unintelligible for ordinary people. The farming out of drug and other forms of medical research to developing countries has always been abused.

Human subject research was one of the few related subjects I rarely wrote about over my career at any length. But what mainly caught my eye were three features of that research that I looked at from a different perspective than was common—one that was much debated and two others that have not been. The debated issue was whether it should be acceptable to use children for research that might help other children eventually but would have no direct benefit for them. Paul Ramsey argued that such a use would be flatly wrong, treating children as means, not ends, to some higher good. The Jesuit theologian Richard McCormick defended such a use, holding that though they could not as children give informed consent, they should be treated as if the ought to wish to consent if they could do so.

I considered McCormick's a poor argument, but I was intrigued by two related features brought out by its critics. Hans Jonas voiced one of them by holding that although medical research was a human good its aim is "melioristic," not obligatory: "Our descendants have the right to be left an unplundered planet; they do not have a right to new miracle cures." Paul Ramsey spoke of McCormick's position as amounting to a "research imperative" that made medical research not merely a good but a moral obligation. Not until many years later did I recall that exchange, nor did others take up and explore the putative obligation to carry out research to which Jonas and Ramsey called attention.

Decades later, in 2003, I published a book to more fully develop the case against a research imperative, *What Price Better Health: Hazards of the Research Imperative*. Medical research is a human good, not an ethical obligation. It should be treated to the same kind of analysis about its opportunity costs (are there other and possibly better ways of spending money?) as other human goods. It is no less important to recognize that to turn research into a moral imperative is to invite it to run roughshod over other ethical considerations—exactly what happened with the Tuskegee research.

The other two issues that attracted my attention were the IRBs' lack of authority to question the medical goals of human subject research or its possible social harm. A potential research subject can use his or her freedom of consent to raise objections to the goals of the research and to question its value, and also to refuse to take part. But the IRB itself can do that only in cases where the goals seem flagrantly trivial or pose risks well beyond their potential health benefits. Only the protection of research subjects is within the scope of their authority. I came to think of this as the ends and means problem, most notable with some later government commissions (e.g., a National Academy of Sciences study of stem cell research) that did not raise ethical objections but took for granted that those objections had already been met and their goal now is to make sure the chosen means to carry out the research are acceptable. Perhaps the comparison is excessive, but it is as if the ethics of capital punishment turns only on the right of the condemned to spiritual counsel, a last meal of their own choice, and a clean set of clothes.

The other interesting feature of human subject research is the uncommonly high moral status given to informed consent. As autonomy became a dominant value in American bioethics, its protection in human subject research became its capstone. As a principle it would admit no compromise for competent adult subjects, even if the research promised to save a life. Nor does it admit any overriding research imperative, that is, no individual moral obligation to be a research participant. Even those who argue that there is a moral obligation to take part in clinical trials, none do so by contending that the obligation entails a duty to give up their right to refuse consent. To make that argument would bring down the whole edifice of ethical human subject research.

## Autonomy and Responsibility

What stands out as unique about the absolutist status given to informed consent was that autonomy in other contexts moved the field in exactly the opposite direction, toward a libertarianism sometimes little removed from sheer moral relativism. That trend in itself would hardly be surprising in American culture, putting a high value on the right to choose one's own direction in life and to make use of technology to do so. More disturbing was another feature of that trend: using autonomy as a way of evading moral responsibility. Despite it being rarely enunciated as such, there is what I would call an principle of responsible choice if there is to be morality at all: as individuals, we are morally responsible for the reasonably foreseeable consequences of our autonomous choices and actions. I will cite the three examples in which I believe that autonomy has been used to evade the principle: the tethered violinist thought experiment, sperm and egg donation, and efforts to enhance human traits and capacities.

In a much-cited 1970 article on abortion in *Philosophy and Public Affairs*, MIT philosopher Judith Jarvis Thompson asked us to imagine the following situation: waking up to find that tethered to us is a violinist who will die if deprived of the life support his connection to us makes possible. Thompson contends that we would have no obligation to allow that situation to continue, even if breaking off the connection means the death of the violinist. Analogously, no woman has an obligation to use her body to maintain the life of an unplanned and unwanted fetus. Her basic principle to ground that contention is that we are responsible for only those choices we voluntarily enter into. She does not deny that it would be a worthy act of beneficence to allow the line to be left in place to save the life but that, strictly speaking, it is not obligatory. So also with the unplanned fetus. The attractiveness of this line of argument is that it altogether bypasses the moral status of the fetus. She does not deny the value of the life of the violinist; it is just that the situation relieves us of responsibility for that life.

I never found her argument persuasive, if only because her thought experiment is not at all analogous to that of sexual relationships. It can work well enough in circumstances of rape or otherwise coerced sex, but not when there is sex between "consenting adults," as a common legal phrase puts it. If consenting means that (a) the choice is voluntary and (b) one is aware that unprotected sex carries with it a high probability of pregnancy and that not all contraceptives are 100 percent reliable, then the principle of moral responsibility applies. It is a choice, the consequences of which are reasonably foreseeable.

The fact that a woman in that circumstance does not want to get pregnant is ethically beside the point. She has put herself knowingly in a vulnerable situation, taking a known risk. To claim a lack of responsibility for the outcome is to violate the moral principle that goes with claims of autonomy. To reject the Thompson argument is hardly to reject other ways of defending abortion (and even she does not claim that it deals with all objections), but I would characterize it as a misuse of the idea of autonomy given what is knowable about sexual choices. Analogously, a judge would reject the plea of a prisoner to be free of a drunk driving charge and resulting accident on the grounds that although he knew of the dangers of driving inebriated but did his best to drive slowly and carefully, he surely did not intend for the accident to happen.

My second example is that of sperm and egg donation, particularly when it is anonymous. Very simply put, a person who donates the sperm or egg that is used to cause a pregnancy is the biological parent of a resulting child. If the donation were made to bring about the procreation as a reasonably foreseeable outcome, the donor has the same moral responsibility for the future welfare of the resulting child as if the procreation was the deliberate act of a couple who wanted to share its biological heritage.

It is precisely the denial of that responsibility that is a violation of the moral axiom of autonomy. By legally allowing such donations, especially when anonymous, society has done no less than set aside by fiat a basic moral responsibility of deliberate parenthood. It eliminates responsibility altogether. And it is all the worse when some sperm donors are the fathers of many children, who are then related to each other. But does not legal adoption, where responsibility for the welfare of a child is legally trans- ferred to a person or a couple who is willing to take it over, violate the axiom also? The difference is that typically in the instance of adoption, the biological parents are unable to discharge their duties, putting their child at risk; even then, there has been a movement in recent years to allow adopted children to find out who their biological parents are. A small but growing international effort (led by children so procreated) is underway to allow donors to be identified if desired, and by a smaller group, to have egg and sperm donation to be made illegal (though how this could done effectively is uncertain).

### How Important Is the Biological Relationship?

What value should be assigned to a genetic relationship between parent and child? Three different perspectives can be discerned. One of them is that a genetic relationship between parent and children is irrelevant. What counts is the quality of the relationship, one that should be marked by love, affection, and a commitment to the welfare of the child. The bond between adopted children and their adopting parents can be as strong and real as when a genetic connection exists. Another view is that for many would-be parents, a genetic connection is important, out of a belief that the parent-child bond will be stronger than with an adopted child or will help to hold on to a family lineage, or that it is somehow more "natural." A third view is that because there is no good way to choose between the first and second options, either choice is acceptable and should be legally sanctioned. There is a paradox, even a kind of contradiction, here: those who support donation stress the irrelevance of a biological connection for the donor-child relationship while affirming its importance for the person who wants the donation in order to have that relationship. That is, to have it both ways.

My position is that to allow sperm or egg donation without a cor- responding acceptance of a parental obligation of the donor to the child's welfare is a misuse of the value of autonomy, a violation of personal responsibility. A system in which there were no anonymous donors and an agreement that in times of need or crisis, the donor would be obliged to accept full responsibility, would be a different and perhaps acceptable policy.

## The Lure of Enhancement

My third case is that of efforts to enhance human traits or capabilities. I reject at the outset one way simply to make the ethical problem go away. It is to deny there is any difference in principle between corrective improvements in human life (e.g., eyeglasses or surgery for congenital heart defects) that ordinary medical progress has brought about and more deliberate efforts to significantly go beyond those possibilities to radically improve human life or extend a functioning life. A common example offered to support the notion is that there is no inherent difference between vaccination, which enhances the body's resistance to germs and viruses, and efforts (still speculative) to double average human IQ. But even in the most lethal plagues, most people will not catch the disease or die from it—only those with some susceptibility. A vaccine brings those with the susceptibility up to the ordinary standard of natural resistance. That strategy is not inherently different than providing a prosthetic device to allow someone with an amputated leg to walk again. Indeed, most medicine aims not to create some new trait or capacity but to restore what has been lost by illness or accident or to help those born with genetic or other abnormalities to be brought as near to an ordinary life as possible.

That much said, I mean by "enhancement" the effort to improve human life well beyond the present levels of capacity for either populations as a whole or individuals. That enhancement may aim for greatly increased memory or intelligence, a removal of tendencies to destructive violence, much improved endurance for athletic or other purposes, or a radical increase in average life expectancy (one claim is the possibility of a 2,500-year life span). The greatest ethical obstacle to pursuing such goals is the impossibility of reliably and responsibly projecting the long-term social and individual consequences of such goals. The violation of the responsibility principle comes in when, in the name of freedom of choice, enhancement is sought without any way of knowing whether it will turn out as hoped and whether it can be turned back when it comes out badly. In that case, it would be foolish to embark upon it in the first place.

That some individuals aspire to enhancement, either for themselves or in their research in behalf of others, seems to be accepted as a sufficient reason to go forward. The exercise of autonomy in this case turns simply on the desire to use it, not on the moral value of the ends themselves. The standard for responsible autonomy should be the need for enhancement in the first place or for its likelihood of bringing individual benefits without doing social harm. By a "need" for enhancement, I mean the possibility that it will relieve some present human or social deficiency, such as that of the relief of pain and suffering, poverty, war and destructive social distress, everyday crime and violence, or a failure of people to achieve their possible capabilities. But a lack of high IQs has never been identified as a cause of those ills—most tyrannical dictators and genocidal leaders do not lack high intelligence, they just used it wrongly—nor would an improvement in the average human memory have any sure benefits in life (our ability over time to forget our troubles is a blessing not a curse).

A radical extension of life expectancy has nothing to be said for it of social merit. No present social harm comes from an average life expectancy of 78, our present American level, nor would it if it had stopped at 75—and it is far from clear that the average age of 85 for Japanese women has given them inherently better lives than they had when it was 75. In fact, the great Japanese worry is that with an extremely low birthrate, the added years may consist of greater misery for lack of adequate resources to pay for those additional years. In short, the fantasies of enhancement require an abnegation of responsibility to pursue them, given that we cannot predict their benefit, and a failure of imagination to envision how they could all go wrong.

Yet a proviso is that if one can assemble sufficient evidence from existing or past ways of life that show a safe and successful precedent for the enhancement, then that may justify going forward. Greater choice and control by themselves, to echo Joseph Fletcher as cited above, do not assure real human progress. They can just as well be their enemy. The gambler's principle is not a wise or prudent principle when trying to change human beings.

## Parental Obligations

A more immediate example of efforts to use autonomy as a rationale for changing our human biology is that of choosing the genetic or other traits of our children, either pre- or postnatally. The right to choose whether to have children, and to decide on their timing, was a good and legitimate cause for the family planning movement. It did not take long, however, for that freedom of procreation to be extended in the name of autonomy to choose the sex and other traits of our children, that is, to have the kind of children we want, not the kind that the chance and vagaries of uncontrolled procreation give us. The first step down that road was the moral legitimation of abortion to avoid defective or otherwise damaged children, assumed to be a benefit to the aborted child but even more clearly a benefit to parents who did not want that kind of child. The kind of child one is likely to become is seen as morally legitimate a consideration as whether to have children at all.

Although it is surely understandable that parents would prefer not to have severely handicapped children, it seems to me incredibly naïve for them to think that either they or their child will be happier or made better off if they can control the sex or other important traits of their children to somehow have an improved, higher-grade child. Here is a good example of an aspiration about which there is much ordinary evidence lying at hand to question its wisdom: the resentment that children feel against excessively pushy parents, loving the child of one sex rather than another for that reason alone, and the often mistaken disappointment of parents when their children eventually choose religions or careers or ways of life that thwart parental ambitions. King Lear learned about such mistakes the hard way.

A 14-year-old friend of my granddaughter says that she hates her physician father for wanting her to go to the Harvard Medical School, nastily criticizing her for getting less than an A+ in every course, and forcing her to take (in the eighth grade!) a tutorial class for her future SATs. Tennis star Andre Agassiz said in his autobiography that he never forgave his parents for coercing him into the sport.

I readily concede that much of this evidence is anecdotal and that there is a fine line to be walked here. What about mothers famous for their powerful role in shaping their children—for instance, the mothers of St. Augustine, Franklin D. Roosevelt, Andrew Carnegie, and Douglas

MacArthur? And was there anything wrong when, after four sons, we hoped for (and got) a girl? Most parents want to have children who will be happy, successful in the life they choose, morally good in their behavior, and a credit to their love and sacrifice in raising them.

But the enhancement question is this: to what extent and in what ways is it morally legitimate to attempt to procreate and raise children with traits that reflect more the parental desires than the welfare of the child, or who fail to see the difference between those aims? The paradox of procreation is that people want children for the pleasure and satisfaction they can bring to their lives, but they will be in trouble as parents if they forget the even greater importance of the pleasure and satisfaction they should aim for in the lives of those children, their first duty. In any case, children rarely satisfy fully their parents' dreams and sometimes, to their dismay and best efforts, become bad dreams as the child's life turns out, or sometimes become alienated and distant in their adulthood from even fine parents for often inexplicable reasons.

The sex of a child is no predictive indicator of that child's temperament and congeniality, its intelligence or social sensibilities, its love of its parents. The lottery of procreational luck is likely to be as good as any designer children, and is a psychologically better preparation for parenthood, that of raising children who will have to make their own lives apart from their parents.

What became evident by the 1980s in any case was that medical research and practice would put before parents many new choices and possibilities, a good number of them nearly impossible to evade once various kinds of knowledge and technology became available. Whether parents like it or not, the social pressure to move in one direction or the other is increasingly inescapable. When prenatal diagnosis became available in the 1960s, its use was introduced as simply a new and potentially valuable free choice for parents. But there is a good historical rule of thumb to remember when a new technology is said to be wholly voluntary: it may begin that way but will probably become routine by habituation and social pressure.

## The Drift of Choice to Social Coercion

By the 1980s, prenatal diagnosis was becoming routine for pregnant women, socially sanctioned, and then as routinized as the taking of blood pressure; social pressure amounting to coercion had done its work. It is not impossible to reject it, but doing so is not much easier than deciding to take a horse to work rather than a car—a real choice a century ago. The same will be true of prenatal and postnatal screening for later life disease threats. The transhumanists, who think we are on the edge of taking over our evolutionary future (a growing number), seem inveterately incapable of imagining the possibility of either technological disasters or the coercive force of new and popular technologies, potently aided by so-called market freedom, to enslave us. The power of technological innovation to overpower doubt and resistance is enormous.

I have in the preceding few pages blurted out a variety of opinions that many will agree with and many will not. They reveal, not far below the surface, a wariness of technology, a sharp eye for the shortcomings of autonomy, particularly in its libertarian strain, and what many will take to be old-fashioned conservatism in my criticisms of sperm and egg donation. Am I here showing, with the donation issue, vestiges of my earlier Catholicism or, equally plausible, a leftover remnant of the technology-wary liberalism of the 1960s and the legacy of Hiroshima and Nagasaki, which left a profound mark on my 15-year-old psyche in 1945?

Possibly so in the latter case, but I raise those questions because, by the 1980s, an earlier generation of scientists, often trained in Europe, who had organized the conferences of the 1960s to discuss the potential harms as well as benefits of the "biological revolution," had begun dying out. In their place came a new generation, less interested in ethical and political matters and under pressure to steer clear of them in order to not harm their chances of getting grants, which had become more competitive. And although it is hard to know what the long-term impact on American medicine would be, by the end of the 1970s there was a decisive move by some leading scientists into economic entrepreneurship, rejecting a long history of looking down their noses at such crass behavior.

By then, some of the friends and supporters of the Center were worried that the very process of critically examining new medical and biological technologies could "give the wrong impression" to potential donors. There was some basis in our journals and project reports for such worries. And we worried a bit about the worries, not because we felt we had gone out of our way to be skeptical about commonly trumped medical breakthroughs but because it seemed unavoidable. If we were to be serious about ethics, it was necessary to look for the potential downside of technological developments as fully and openly as the enthusiastic proponents sought to paint the brightest possible pictures. We live in a society that tilts the less-than-level playing field toward acceptance, not rejection, of technology. At the same time, and on a parallel course, various critics chastised us for taking money from pharmaceutical companies, even though there were never any strings attached. Or so we thought. On two occasions, the hand that (partly) fed us (Pfizer and Eli Lilly) abruptly withdrew their annual grants when we published articles they found objectionable—and they let us know that was the reason.

## The Pluralism Puzzle

If the problem of ethical theory and the foundations of ethics and bio-ethics had been important for the first generation of bioethicists, two new struggles surfaced in the 1980s: competing notions of ethical theory and cultural pluralism. Two were particularly important: feminism and contextualism. As they had done in many other arenas, a number of feminists accused the field of bias against women, by its failure to call attention to the way women were treated in medical care and by its unwillingness to take account of imbalances of power in its ethical theory.

It was not—and still is not—hard to find solid data showing that there was a differential in the treatment of males and females in health care: women were often treated in a patronizing and demeaning way, less attention was paid to their wishes, and men were more likely to have beneficial, even life-saving treatment than women. We had no doubt that the charges were correct and the conduct indefensible. Moreover, the rationalistic moral theories of ethics bore the markings of a male picture of the role of reason and emotion. Carol Gilligan of the Harvard School of Education attracted considerable attention for her studies showing that women were more likely than men to take an interpersonal rather than an impersonal and principle- and rule-driven approach to moral dilemmas. Along the way, she rejected the work of Lawrence Kohlberg, which posited different stages of moral development, from gross self-interest at the bottom ("don't get caught") to an embrace of altruistic justice at the top.

Kohlberg did not have many bioethicists among his followers, but Gilligan's work did have some influence. That influence came to blend in almost indistinguishable ways with contextualism, which also—against rules and principles—stressed the importance of social and personal context and culture in the framing and solution of ethical problems. Joseph Fletcher had more or less said the same some decades earlier with his espousal of situation ethics (known to philosophers as a version of act utilitarianism—rejecting general rules and principles in favor of judging the consequences of each moral action). What attracted attention was the perception in both cases that the generality and abstractness of classical ethical theory simply did not and could not take account of the social and cultural imbedded nature of moral judgments, a complaint also lodged against bioethics by social scientists.

For me, someone who had from my earliest graduate school days been wary of high-level moral theory and later of principlism, the feminist-contextualist perspective was congenial and helpful. But the feminist charges against physicians and medical practice were another matter, having nothing to do with their validity, which seemed undeniable. The larger question for me as director of the Hastings Center was whether and to what extent our work on ethics should encompass campaigns or crusades against patent wrong-doing.

That problem was a dilemma for an organization that was established to study ethical problems of medicine and biology, taking stands now and then with its research, but not to be a whistle-blowing outfit against any and all medical evils. On the one hand, the kinds of abuses uncovered by Henry K. Beecher in the gross misuse of human research subjects and the revelations of the lethal Tuskegee abuses demanded ethical reform and regulation. On the other hand, over the years we received a steady stream of personal stories or news reports of all kinds of other abuses: physician sexual misconduct with patients or verbal abuse by doctors of nurses, tales of fraudulent Medicare claims, dangerous hospital practices, and racial, gender, and age bias.

### What Are the Moral Duties of an Ethics Research Center?

In most cases, there was little disagreement that the perpetrations of those actions were wrong and directly in contravention of the law or medical codes of ethics. But should we take them all on? Another group of critics said that the transcendent evil was inequitable health care, far worse than the precious fussing about such issues as physician misconduct, human cloning, enhancement possibilities, and transgender operations. We were irresponsible for not throwing our full weight against that atrocity. I came to think of that latter critique as a piece of ethical one-upmanship: whatever issues we took up were always trumped by still higher, more important issues. And one early critic attacked us for worrying about ethics and medicine when the real problem, he vehemently said, was the Arab-Israeli conflict. Others identified poverty in the developing world as the overriding evil and asked: why were we dodging that one?

We thus had to sort our views about where to place our emphasis and also, simultaneously, to determine what it meant for us to claim, as we did (and do), to be neutral and nonpartisan in a field supercharged with arguments and ideological riptides as we did so. Although we did not develop written rules to deal with these various problems, some informal rules of thumb were gradually shaped. Others were already taking on abuse and global health problems, and in any event, our issues were important even if, from a global perspective, not necessarily the most important. As for the stream of requests that we take on, investigate, and rectify the lesser but real misbehaviors to be found in medicine, we had and have no investigative skills or capacities. More important was that our work was best focused, we believed, on the moral problems and dilemmas posed by medical advances instead of on patently wrong and well-recognized illegal and immoral behavior. The fact of harmful fraud in the Medicare program presented a moral problem easier to deal with than the ethical allocation of scarce resources to the old.

Is it really possible to be nonpartisan? Not entirely. Our requirement for the organization of research projects was that the opposing positions on controversial issues had to be taken seriously and presented with fairness. Our research groups were free to come to conclusions about ethical and policy problems, but they had to be presented in a way that clearly showed a serious effort to take account of other views. The arguments presented in favor of a position had to be plausible, even if they would be judged wrong by many. But if our research groups and articles we published could take strong stands, the Center as an institution took (and still takes) no stands at all. We had agreed from the start that in a field full of legal, ethical, and social disagreements, our best contribution would be as an honest broker, working to speak in a civil tone, respecting the various actors, and doing what we could to bring some illumination to murky and often impossibly hard problems.

Inevitably, however, it was possible for critics of another ideological stripe to discern a liberal bias in our work and publications. I say "inevitably" for two reasons. The most obvious was that most of our journal contributors and board members have been liberal, at least in a procedural way, upholding the importance of not using a person's moral bias as a reason for rejecting articles or convictions expressed in conference reports. If hardly in every issue, readers of the *Hastings Center Report* can expect that over a period of time, major ethical debates will receive a full airing and diverse voices heard.

## The Liberal Bias

The other reason was that most of those recruited have been academics and scientific researchers, and they are as a group mostly secular or liberal in their religious belief, that is, fairly representative of American intellectuals and scholars. We have had no hesitations about publishing conservative articles, for instance, but comparatively few over the years have been submitted to us, and they were as likely to be accepted as any others. As the culture wars accelerated in the late 1990s and at the turn of the millennium, it became evident that many conservatives saw liberal bioethics as an enemy to be combated. There would be no fraternizing with that enemy, no presentation of both sides of a controverted issue in their journals, and few efforts to work out compromise solutions.

Many liberals of course shared some of the same kind of zeal in opposition to conservative stands, but they were proportionately fewer in number within the liberal ranks and always a problem for us when they crossed the line between strong, but carefully wrought, positions and intemperate liberal bigotry. Although it is doubtless an overgeneralization, I think liberals have been drawn to bioethics because they see cultural and moral disarray, some of it their own doing, as creating historically new ethical problems. Conservatives, in contrast, see the moral disarray but feel called to defend ancient values and traditions that they often consider under assault by liberals.

I have gone into more detail about these internal struggles than might be interesting or worth knowing, but I have done so to indicate that we have tried to take seriously the question of how an organization devoted to examining ethical problems should behave ethically in the process. We have believed that an open and serious democratic dialog is necessary for coping legally and politically with them; so how ought we to talk and sound? Those have been perennial questions for us. And despite all the uncomplimentary words I have voiced about the training in analytic philosophy I received, I am glad for the rigor it demanded in ethical and philosophical analysis; however, no less did I learn from the Socratic dialogs what it is like to fully pursue a problem in a way that is a serious exchange between two fellow human beings: respectful, relentlessly probing, altogether civilized.

While struggles were breaking out along liberal and conservative lines, they were overshadowed by the issue of pluralism. The publication in 1981 of *After Virtue: A Study in Moral Theory* by philosopher Alasdair MacIntyre was important for its bold thesis. Moral philosophy and western culture more generally, he argued, had failed in the aftermath of the eighteenth-century Enlightenment to replace the virtue ethics of Aristotle, coherent in content and influential in combination with Christianity for centuries thereafter. "The project of providing a rational vindication of morality had decisively failed," MacIntyre wrote, "and from henceforward the morality of our predecessor culture—and subsequently our own lacked any public, shared rationale or justification." In particular, it cut the ground out of "a liberal individualist point of view."

For philosophy, he added, that meant a "loss of its central cultural role and becoming a marginal, narrowly academic subject." We have been left with merely the fragments of a more coherent virtue-based Aristotelian ethics (but which also required a counterpart morality of rules).

H. Tristram Englehardt, Jr., came to a similar conclusion, holding than "a deliberative democracy that would reflect the demands of a canonical bioethics established by sound rational argument cannot in principle be realized."

The feminist embrace of contextualism was meant as a response to the shortcomings of the rationalistic foundations of liberal individualism. But feminism has never had behind it a well-developed social ethic other than equality for women and the same opportunities in life as men have, all of which require an overthrow of patriarchal cultures. But too often in the end that comes down to simply an ethic of individualist choice, not only with abortion decisions but with most other significant moral decisions as well. The accompanying contextualism did not help. If anything, it invited the omission of a consideration of what a good life may require—which moral choices are good and bad—which contexts alone rarely are capable of revealing. Neither did it offer a way of judging the validity of the background social and political culture that shapes the social particularities that produce the context for making ethical decisions. If a rationalistic liberalism could find no ethical core, the antidote of personalized contextualism does not work to fill the gap.

## The Advent of John Rawls

By the 1980s, a generation of philosophers and political scientists educated under the influence of John Rawls's 1971 book *A Theory of Justice* had begun writing on health care using Rawls's theory as their point of departure. It is an elegantly argued book, but it's also notable for its deliberate unwillingness to apply the theory to issues as specific as health care. That was left for his followers to do, and many took up the challenge—notably, Norman Daniels (then at Tufts, now at Harvard) in his 1985 book *Just Health Care*. But I had trouble getting caught up in the enthusiasm. Rawls begins his case for his theory of justice with a "thought experiment," which I considered then and now the worst and irreducibly most slack way of pursuing philosophical knowledge. He posited what a person behind a veil of ignorance would think about justice, not knowing where he might personally be in terms of intelligence, social class, and individual talents. Behind that veil, the rational person would a view of justice that promised equal opportunity to achieve the necessities of life, where what benefited the well off would also have to benefit the least well off, and whose free choices in life would be equal to everyone else's free choices.

I hardly do justice to the nuances of Rawls's theory, but I wonder why he chose such a dubious starting point. He might more profitably have spent many of the years he took writing that book to travel around the world as an anthropologist or psychologist might, inductively gathering what different cultures and modes of thought and emotion made of the concept, rooting justice in human experience. Instead, his kind of thought experiment was based in the end on a highly individualistic way of looking at the world, how a fully rational but otherwise detached person would think (shades of an "ideal observer theory"). But for his followers, that meant a move from an individualistic premise to a communitarian conclusion, which to me is in the same category as putting square blocks in round holes. For that and a variety of other reasons, I have never believed that good arguments for justice as the moral foundation for health care are persuasive, nor that theories of a right to health care work.

Quite apart from the obvious fact that justice- and rights-based theories have never over fifty years of health reform debate gained much public and legislative traction in the United States and are hardly invoked in European health care either (where the concept of solidarity is most commonly used), the ideological split between right and left over the years has revealed very different ways in which ideological differences play themselves out in politics. The steady, near 50/50 split over fifty years or so between liberals and conservatives on health care reform regarding whether it should be government- or a market-oriented showed as well as anything could that in actual life—and with the same general evidence before their eyes—people can have fundamentally different judgments about what will be good for them and what kind of chances they are prepared to take with their lives. Only hypothetical rational calculators behind a hypothetical screen are likely to come out with such a tidy consensus on fairness as Rawls and Norman Daniels and other care reformers did, following Rawls's lead. But, having said that, I have profited from reading both of them.

I will note that in 1975, I was the chairman of the National Book Award for nonfiction and had worked to get the committee to award the prize to the libertarian colleague of Rawls, Robert Nozick. My colleagues on the committee objected to his political philosophy, as did I, but I made the successful case that Nozick's considerable philosophical skills, not his conclusions, should be our only criterion for judgment. But Nozick's facility with argument, as well as drawing from a long libertarian tradition that put freedom before justice, showed that what people can want outside of a veil of ignorance can be as rational as what they might choose behind it and can simply go in a different direction than toward justice. Many Americans—perhaps as many as half—believe they have no obligation to pay taxes to help the uninsured, or much empathy for them either. Arguments about justice have no power at all with them. Detailed stories and extensive data about the economic and physical suffering of those without insurance, or the poor more generally, are exceedingly rare in the *Wall Street Journal*.

### Euthanasia and Physician-Assisted Suicide

Sporadically during this period, efforts in the states to change laws against euthanasia and physician-assisted suicide (PAS) began to pick up after many futile efforts going back to the 1930s. The Netherlands was becoming known as a country in which, though the law still forbade them, the courts were making decisions freeing from prosecution physicians who took part in them. By the late 1980s and into the 1990s, those efforts accelerated in the United States all the more, stimulated by Dr. Kevorkian's illegal freelance efforts, Derek Humphry and the Hemlock Society, and a steady stream of articles and news stories. Public opinion surveys of physicians and laymen usually showed a slightly favorable majority.

Although it is surely easy to understand why euthanasia and PAS would be desired by some, a perfectly attractive idea in the face of the assorted miserable ways people can die, I have always opposed it. This position may seem odd given the various other beliefs I hold. I believe it is morally acceptable for competent patients to ask that life-extending treatment be terminated, that sustaining the life of someone in a persistent vegetative state with continued food and water is useless and should not be done, and that it makes sense for someone whose inevitable death is on the way to stop eating and taking water. Conservatives who oppose at least some of those possibilities mistakenly conflate the sanctity of life as a moral principle and the technological imperative as a de facto rule of aggressive medical care; that is, what can be done technologically to extend life ought to be done.

The stumbling block for me is that of the empowerment of physicians to either directly kill patients (euthanasia) or to assist patients to take their own lives (PAS). Suicide is no longer illegal in the United States, and thus patients are free to commit suicide; that would be a legally acceptable autonomous choice. But to use the social authority of medicine and physicians to legitimate euthanasia and PAS would be to sully the traditional role of doctors and to invite abuse. Doctors are much more proficient than the rest of us in knowing how to bring about death, and the experience of the Netherlands over the years as revealed by anonymous surveys turned up a large number—more than 1,000 per year—of physicians killing their patients without gaining their assent.

The hospice movement and improved palliative care obviate most of the claimed need to use death to cure pain. But physical pain is not the main reason for a use of PAS and euthanasia. Surveys in both the Netherlands and, more recently, Oregon have revealed that most of those who want either of them do so because of a loss of control over their lives, a diminishment of their chosen way life—that is, their motive is one of a loss of a desired lifestyle, not because of physical pain and the ordinary anguish of dying. Only in the most trivial sense is there any loss of human dignity in even a very bad death. The small number of patients in Oregon who have chosen PAS—more than 400 in its first decade—suggests that far more people think they would want PAS to relieve their dying than actually do in practice. I should note, in any case, that it is now and has always been possible to for a doctor to give a troubled dying patient potentially lethal pain-relieving drugs and to say nothing more to a patient other than, "Be careful not to take too many of these at once; they could kill you."

## Death: A Technological, Not Biological, Failure

There has always been another ancillary feature of that debate that is important. It has become almost dogma among many bioethicists, particularly the philosophers, that there is no ethical difference between directly killing a patient—say, by a lethal injection—and turning off a ventilator, an action that will no less effectively end a life. One consequence of accepting this belief is that it makes use of already acceptable actions by physicians to show that euthanasia and PAS are no different morally and should thus be accepted.

But there are some untoward implications in moving in that direction. One of them is, in effect, to embrace a view of death in the company of modern medicine which holds that death is no longer a function of what it is happening to the body. It is instead only a failure of technology, wielded by the physician, to sustain life. In short, the doctor is made responsible for all death, whether by direct action or indirectly by terminating treatment. Yet unlike most philosophers, most physicians continue to accept the distinction between killing and allowing to die. Why?

One likely reason is that every doctor knows that, sooner or later, everyone of his or her patients will die, either under his or her care or that of some other physician. The human body ages, declines, and dies. That is the way things are. A physician who terminates life-extending treatment because of its futility and medical uselessness is doing nothing more than recognizing that biological truth. The fact that a patient might have lived on a few more days or weeks with aggressive interventions does not overcome that truth. It makes sense then, as the deniers of the distinction deny, to say that it was the patient's underlying disease that killed the patient, not the doctor. One might as well say that someone who stops shoveling snow from her driveway in a blizzard because she can't keep up with the falling snow is thereby responsible for a driveway full of snow at the end of the storm. Death can overcome even the best treatment, just as a big enough storm can overcome the best shoveler.

A final note here. I have come to wonder what kind of moral model, so to speak, a dying person should be to those around him or her if that is possible. The dying patient will be cared for by physicians and nurses, families, and friends, who will someday be in the same situation themselves. What kind of memory of us would we like them to have when their time comes? I would say such a thing of someone who tried to accept death, who tried not to be self-pitying and to be as cheerful and brave as possible, and who is above all sensitive and responsive to and thankful for the help others were providing, which is often emotionally painful.

Many of those with far more experience than I have in caring for the dying have told me that people seem to bring to their deathbed the same personality and emotional traits they had all their lives: whiners whine, the self-centered note only their own suffering and seem indifferent to the help others are trying to provide. My model was Dan Clouser, a pioneer bioethicist at Penn State. He was a funny, sociable, and much loved person. When I saw him (all ninety pounds of him) in a hospital a week or so before his death from a five-year struggle with cancer of the pancreas, he had the medical staff laughing at his resolute humor and good spirits, just as he had done with everyone else when he was in good health.

## Assessing Rationalizations

There is still one other ethical problem raised by that debate, one that is related to an earlier mentioned issue and that will come up again later. It might be called the *rationalization problem* or, more colloquially put, a variant of the chicken-and-egg problem of ethics. Is the motive of those who believe there is no distinction between killing and allowing to die that of opening the door to euthanasia, which it does, or can it stand as an independent judgment accepted for its own sake regardless of its bearing on euthanasia? Is the motive of doctors who accept the distinction an unwillingness to tolerate the possibility that every patient who dies under their care is because of their own doing, even if we do not want to say that it is their fault? Is it a coincidence that most pro-choice advocates believe that the embryo and fetus have a low moral status, thus making abortion more easily defensible, or that pro-life advocates believe in its high moral status, thus making abortion more acceptable?

To this day, I cannot say whether the less-than-fully-a-person status I attributed to embryos and fetuses was an unrecognized function of the sympathy for women's plight I developed during my research, or whether the sympathy came more easily once I had decided that the embryo or fetus were not full persons and thus had a lower standing. Nor could I be certain that I did not adopt the distinction between the beginning of life and the beginning of personhood, which makes at least early abortion easier to accept, because I was looking for a moral way to legitimate it. I wonder about that to this day, uncertain whether it is a valid distinction. How do we answer such questions about our motives, and do they matter anyway? To "know thyself" is not so easy in ethics, and I don't know myself well enough to be sure I came to the right judgment. But then I am not certain that certainty is where we should ever come out with regard to problems that seem inherently hard. And I am not certain whether that is the right way to think about our solutions, either. Sometimes I just end up wringing my hands, worn out as much from arguing with myself as with others.

# 5

## The Routinization of Charisma: 1986–1996

The "routinization of charisma" is a wonkish phrase, not to be used in polite company. But there is no better way to describe a classic problem with startup companies or think tanks. They begin with a great splash and move with a fast, exciting pace. Then the excitement wears off, the entrepreneurial leaders get short of breath and fresh ideas, and an orderly long-term routine must be put in place.

After charisma, then what? By the mid-1980s, that was our situation. We were well established, solid enough to run an endowment campaign, and working at a fast and often exhausting pace. The circulation of the *Hastings Center Report* was 10,500, much larger than that of any other bioethics journal. Our influential work in Eastern Europe was just beginning, and we received all the media attention anyone could want. We lost many of our early stars to medical schools and universities starting their own programs (and usually paying higher salaries). That was troublesome, but flattering in a way. We had recruited them because of their unusual promise and their willingness to take a chance with a new organization in a new field that offered no tenure or security. Many of the leaders now in the field started with us as staff members or interns. I was sorry to see them go, but proud that they had made their name with us.

Bioethics itself was rapidly moving into its own routinization of charisma. The interest of government in bioethics was both a sign of the status of bioethics and a response to the steady stream of controversial issues that the medical developments were generating. Five federal commissions were initiated by different presidential administrations, beginning with the 1974–1978 National Commission for the Protection of Human Subjects and continuing up to 2009 when President Obama established another commission. That pattern, of new commissions every few years, has been different from the pattern emerging in Europe: setting up government committees as permanent advisory and regulatory bodies.

I was, however, becoming uneasy with the direction of the field, which was moving away from what we originally had in mind. By choosing to be outside of a university and aiming to speak to both a professional and lay audience, we wanted to have a strong public voice but also to show that our work was respectable for scholars in the field. That worked well enough for the first decade or so. But more and more people were drawn into the field, almost all of them academics, and courses on bioethics were proliferating at both the undergraduate and professional levels. The field was drifting toward what it is now—an academic subspecialty.

The typical curriculum vitae (CV) was gradually changing as well. A distinction was made in CVs that we had never made earlier: between peer-reviewed articles professional journals and (allegedly) lower-status publications such as op-ed pieces. (But just try getting an op-ed accepted by the *New York Times*, which I have done only three times, with many more rejections—I have a much better batting average with the *New England Journal of Medicine*.) Despite muttering about it as director of the Hastings Center, I was persuaded by the editors of the *Hastings Center Report* that they had to advertise the fact that it was a peer-reviewed journal, not merely a general interest magazine, in order to get the best people in the field. Between the pressures on academics in the field to publish in peer-reviewed journals and our willingness to make sure we were one of them, the *Hastings Center Report* steadily became an academic journal, though with more colorful and shorter pieces than most of the others. Sometimes as much as 10 percent of any issue was (and is even now) given over to footnotes, an indulgence to academic niceties. One result was inevitable: we lost most of our lay readers and became used to our smart nonacademic board members often reporting that most of the articles in the *Hastings Center Report* were too technical and "over their heads." Looking back, I am sorry that I let that drift take place. We surely lost many of our earlier interested lay readers.

Hardly less attractive was the increasing specialization of those in the field. Younger staff members said that they envied the way in the early days the earlier generation could take on a diverse range of issues—from genetics to end-of-life care, to reproductive biology—in the space of a few years. That was not possible for them, they said; there was just too much to know in the different areas of bioethics. I do not believe that to be true, but the virus of academic specialization had been passed along to them. The fact that I have written on many disparate topics and on just about every bioethics issue seems to impress them in some ways, but then, they say, I am different and thus don't really count.

The acceptance by government of bioethics left me uneasy as well. I have no problem with a large and strong federal government, which seems to me necessary in a large and complex country. I favored a universal access, single-payer plan during the 2008–2009 health reform effort. But taking money from the government to work on ethical issues is a different matter. I think it is a fundamental mission of bioethics to raise basic questions about the ends and goals of medical research and progress, not just to deal with the means used to achieve those goals. But none of the federal agencies open to providing grants for work in ethics are willing to do so if the aim of the research is to question a basic premise of that research: that it is a good thing to do.

Under the George W. Bush administration, embryonic stem cell research was stymied by an executive order setting limits on the use of embryonic cells. Those limits were of course highly unpopular with researchers dependent on NIH money. But it would have been utterly impossible for some opponent of that research, even during the Bush years, to get an NIH grant to develop arguments against it. The scientists who pass judgments on proposed research would not allow open opposition to research with such exciting possibilities. And with few exceptions over the years, biomedical researchers (save for getting federal money for embryonic stem cell research) have been able to do what they want to do. The public and Congress believe in research, the researchers want unfettered research, and if the response to a particular kind of research is too controversial, the standard response is to empower a committee to overcome the obstacles. Mild regulation and oversight is the predicable outcome: the research goes on unimpeded.

## Opening a Door: Elder Health Care Costs

By the mid-1980s, I was an entrepreneur who was not just out of breath. I was tired and thinking of leaving. I had accomplished everything I had set out to do, and my life and not just the field had become boringly routinized.

A chance event opened the door for intensified writing and some new directions in my thinking. In 1985 I was invited to serve on a panel organized by the federal Office of Technology Assessment (OTA) on "Health Care Costs and Medical Technology." I was intrigued. I had never written about the elderly, and hardly anyone else in bioethics had written about them, either, in the context of health care costs. I had little knowledge of geriatrics and gerontology, but it was just the kind of topic I liked: virgin territory. I was enthralled by the panel discussions. They were the first sustained look at the future of the Medicare program in the context of fast-developing technologies. They could simultaneously improve the life expectancy and health of the elderly and also push the costs of care to even higher and dangerous levels.

Here was a fundamental tension, between medical progress and health care costs, that has preoccupied me ever since. To deal with that tension well would require that bioethics move away from a heavy focus on rules and principles for decision making, away from a resort to procedural solutions to large-scale policy issues, and away from an unexamined acceptance of a basic premise of American and modern medicine, that of unlimited medical progress. It was not that those ethical strategies and premises were no longer of value; they were and will continue to be. But they are no longer sufficient. They needed new substantive foundations, but not the kinds of foundations sought by the historical search for ethical theory and not the kinds sought by philosophers.

The foundations I began looking for require more of what I think of as insight and understanding than the formulation of rules, principles, and procedures. That kind of an effort means taking on some basic questions of human life and then relating them to appropriate goals for biomedical research and the provision of health care. It means returning to the kind of philosophy embodied in nineteenth-century American philosophy, that of looking at a whole range of human knowledge— history, literature, the social sciences, and cultural studies, for instance— often outside the normal range of later academic bioethics. It also means trying to recover a tradition of wisdom that was mocked and banished in favor of analytic reductionism.

We cannot think about autonomy well without thinking about how as individuals we ought to go about making good rather than bad choices, and what we want to count as a good or bad choice. What kind of a life ought we want to live? We cannot think about justice in health care without asking what kind of medicine in what kind of health care system is most likely to make that a feasible goal. A system based on the ideal of unlimited medical progress at ever-rising costs is a sure route to injustice. We cannot think about sensible goals for medical research at the policy level, or end-of-life care at the clinical level, without confronting the problem of death in human life. Is death the greatest human evil, and should there be an all-out war against death, which has become the norm for research? We cannot think well about procreation without trying to determine what is good for children apart from what parents might desire in the name of procreative freedom. And we cannot think well and fully about health care for the elderly and the future of Medicare without first trying to understand the place of aging as a social and individual phenomenon in the human life cycle.

I would not claim that a consideration of such questions was then and still is absent from bioethics. They are present in bits and pieces but have not had the prominence of the search for some kind of grand ethical theory to undergird the field. There are in any case not the kinds of questions that lend themselves to some overarching theory, if only because some of them bear on how we might best think about our own lives and others on how we might think about a health care system.

But I did not have the ambition of bringing them to the fore when I served on the panel. It started there but then unfolded in my mind over the course of a few years and some three books later. The immediate upshot of my participation in the OTA panel was the opening stage of my revived zest or bioethics, with issues new to bioethics. I took my first steps by writing my first book after a twelve-year gap, a book on the elderly, *Setting Limits: Medical Goals in an Aging Society.* If the OTA panel had made anything self-evident to me it was that the Medicare program would sooner or later be forced to set some limits on health care for the elderly. The trustees of the Medicare program were already projecting well down the road that the program would run out of money, and later projections led to a common conclusion among policy analysts that its long-term survival would require either a doubling of payroll taxes or cutting benefits in half.

## Resistance to Thinking about the Unthinkable

But I quickly discovered two roadblocks to any thought of using costs to determine health care benefits. The first was that in 1965, when Medicare was put in place, Congress had refused (and continues to refuse) to allow costs to be taken into account in determining recipient benefits. The only allowable standard for benefits is that of "reasonable and necessary," an inherently vague phrase. The fact that there are cancer drugs that can cost $30,000 to $90,000 and add only a month or two of longer life, not a cure, cannot be considered. The second roadblock to a consideration of costs was that most, though not all, of the leaders in medical geriatrics and gerontology saw themselves not only as scholars and researchers but also as advocates for the elderly. For years they had worked hard to combat ageism, the stereotyping and often denigration of the elderly. Any consideration of limits, I found, was taken to be nothing less than the worst kind of ageism, as if the elderly were merely a social burden and not worth the high cost of their care. Moreover, to even entertain such a discussion was itself taken to be a sign of bigotry. An interest in saving the program, my aim, simply was not figured in. As the late Robert Butler, the country's leading geriatrician and the first director of the federal National Institute of Aging, once yelled at me in a cab after a TV debate, it is "offensive to even talk of limits in a country as rich as ours."

## For Doctors: A Fearful Topic

Nonetheless, I was fortified for the battle by taking seriously the Medicare projections, which few seemed to care about, and by some surprising support from a few physicians. Quite independent of the OTA experience, I had continually asked physicians for many years what kind of ethical problems they were having that had not been made public. After a number identified care of the elderly as full of ethical dilemmas, I asked them why we had heard so little about that. One answer I got seemed to reflect the thoughts of many: "It's a delicate topic and we're afraid to talk about it." At the same time, the fact of rationing health care for the elderly in the United Kingdom, brought to American attention by Henry Aaron's book *The Painful Prescription* in 1978, did open a slight window for debate. But the main method used in the United Kingdom was hardly likely to commend itself to Americans: covert rationing by tacit agreement among physicians that denial of dialysis and some other high-technology treatments beyond the age of 55 was economically necessary.

*Setting Limits* was the most reviewed, criticized, praised, and best-selling of all my books. It was one of three finalists for the 1987 Pulitzer Prize for nonfiction, which was won by Richard Rhodes for his superb (and more deserving) book *The Making of the Atom Bomb*, which I consider an indispensable examination of ethics and personal conscience. I began my book with a lengthy review of the medical and sociology research on aging, moved on to Medicare projections and other data, and then presented my policy proposal, emphasizing that it was meant to open a debate about the future. I was not proposing an immediate policy. The essence of my argument was that at some point rationing health care of the elderly would be needed, that it should focus on expensive technological treatments of those over 80 (my present age as I write this), but also that enhanced long-term care and economic support would be necessary. My central argument to support the proposal was that by age 79 or 80 most people had lived long enough to have a full life, even if not all desires had been satisfied, that such age was higher than average life expectancy, and that death at that age could be called "natural."

### Resisting the Reciprocal Obligations of Young and Old

I was not surprised at the almost universal rejection of a flat age limit, said to be ageist, misogynist (women live longer than men and thus would be more harmed by an age-based standard), and simply cruel. I was more surprised at the rejection of another point I made, that there is a reciprocal set of obligations between the young and the old: the young have obligations to the old, and old have obligations to the young. The young have an obligation to care for the old (including their Medicare and Social Security support), and an obligation of the elderly is, I argued, to not take excessive resources from the young. That view was roundly condemned: the elderly were owed whatever it took to give them the best possible care. As anyone who pays attention to local school tax debates knows, they almost always feature a few elderly people who say that because they have no children in the schools, they should not be taxed.

A good society, I believe, will help the young become old, but has no obligation to follow technology where it leads to help the old become indefinitely older. The young cannot be expected to pay for an open frontier for the elderly, knowing no boundaries. Have I changed my mind over the years? Only in one respect: I no longer talk of a "natural end to life" but speak of "living a full life," which can be achieved by age 80. I use that phrase because I have often heard it at funerals of the elderly, rarely marked by any sense of tragedy. A full life is one where one has had the opportunity to enjoy most—not necessarily all—of the goods that a human life can bring: education, work, a family raised to adulthood, travel, and physical and psychological pleasure, among others. It is not necessary to have every wish fulfilled to have a satisfying life.

Though I was excoriated and even picketed at times for *Setting Limits,* even most of the harshest critics said that the book should be read. That is all any author can ask for with a controversial thesis, and the book became a standard reference in the literature and research on aging. Twenty-five years later, much of the hostility had dissipated. In 2009 I wrote a blog post for the *New York Times* on rationing care for the elderly, a short version of my earlier argument. It drew a two-day response of 150 comments, some nasty. But at least half agreed me with on the need for limits, and most of the others agreed that there is a problem but didn't like my solution.

Many people predicted that when I got old (I was 56 when *Setting Limits* was published), I would change my tune. I have not (I'm already past the age I used as a baseline, 80), but I now prefer using the economic tool of quality-adjusted-life-years (QALYs) as the criterion for the use of expensive technologies instead of age as the standard. Age-based rationed per se got an entirely bad reception. As an alternative, QALYS a measure of the relationship of expected life expectancy to the quality of the remaining years, which can be used for judging the use of a technology at any age. It is a standard that benefits the young more than the old in general—but by no means always.

Under this criterion, an elderly person will not ordinarily be, but could be, as good a candidate for an expensive procedure as a young person. That is not unjust in the face of limited resources. I rejected the idea, as one critic put it, that the 90-minute-old child and the 90-year-old adult should be treated alike. That view, in the name of total egalitarian justice for different age groups, seems to me untenable. The old have lived a full life and the young have not, and the latter should have preference when resources are short. I have come to embrace that view all the more strongly as I have watched my children move into middle age. I have had my turn, and theirs is still in the making, with many years to go.

**What Will I Do?**

There is an obvious follow-up question: now that you are over 80, are you prepared to give up expensive technological procedures that might save your life? I hope I would do the right thing and decline to proceed. But I think it foolish to predict how I, or almost anyone, will respond to a critical illness in the future—especially one that might, or might not, be a fatal illness, not knowing in advance which it will be, and for which treatment may or may not be outrageously expensive. Yet because of that uncertainty about my own resolve, I do not want to be left with the decision: what might be good for me might not be good for a society straining to provide adequate health care for all. Thus I want my problem to be solved at the policy level by simply denying me care of an expensive kind, using the available resources for those who are younger. By "denial" I mean, say, as a Medicare benefit, leaving me free to buy it with my own resources if I so chose. But I would hope I would not be tempted to harm my wife's future by mortgaging our family money to help me survive.

One of my sons wrote a nice aphorism that he gave me as a present. "A philosopher," he wrote, "is someone capable of having an idea that is not in his own interest." It is entirely possible that some allocation policies will not be in my personal interest. That will not make them wrong policies. The experience of the 1960 dialysis committee in Seattle showed the impossible difficulties of case-by-case committee decisions. To leave the choice up to the private decisions of individual doctors and patients would carry little likelihood of fairness in many cases from a public perspective.

My experience with the *Setting Limits* battle and the response to it over many years—more favorable as time went on—matches an experience I had at the Hastings Center. I had offered a radical proposal to deal with the cost problem in the Medicare program. It was mainly rejected at the time but has become more acceptable with the passing of time (yet it still has a way to go). New ideas take a while to make their mark. Moreover, by taking a position that gradually gained respectability, I showed that for at least for one person, progress could be made with a controversial issue if you wait long enough.

I mentioned earlier in the book how often ethics as a field has been attacked for unresolved controversies and a lack of progress. Many a first-time visitor to our Hastings Center research meetings, whatever the topic, complains that nobody seemed to agree with anyone else and how frustrating that had been. But my response has been that almost all projects start off that way—most of our topics have been controversial or we would not have taken them on in the first place—and that after two to three years of working together, the debate gets sorted out, people change their minds, and progress has almost always been achieved.

I have applied that experience to my own writings. People like me, who live by the pen, can only look upon their writing as the planting of seeds, some of which may not germinate at all, and those that do may take years to bear fruit. I think that happened with *Setting Limits*. So too do many other difficult ethical problems get solved, even if takes years. To "solve" an ethical problem for policy purposes does not require unanimity of agreement. It is sufficient if it can reach a stage where it commands majority support sufficient to allow tolerable laws and policies to be drawn up—but always leaving open the possibility that new knowledge and ways of thinking may force a change of opinion. Consider some now-conventional principles. Care at the end of life requires respect for a patient's views. Human subject research requires informed consent. Patients have a right to information about their treatment and doctors have the duty to provide it. There is an obligation to relieve pain. The truth should be told to patients. Forty-two years ago, as the Hastings Center was being formed, there was no general medical agreement on any of those propositions. We have moved along.

## The Unconstrained Pursuit of Progress

It took at least 25 years for some (and only that) acceptance of limits on health care for the elderly, so I am not sure how many it will take to get a serious debate going on medical progress, something I have tried to stimulate with a notable lack of success. Medical progress and health care for the elderly are inherently open-ended, as good an example of science as an "endless frontier" as one can find. Their situation can be likened to the exploration of outer space: no matter how far one goes, one could always go further. The evidence is now solid that there is no way of predicting how high average life expectancy can go or how long an individual can live. Japanese women live to an average age of 85, the highest in the world, and then there are also people living beyond 110, approaching the record 122 of a French woman some years ago. But those longer lives are accompanied by the inevitably higher costs of health care for them, intensified in recent decades by the capacity of medicine to keep chronically ill elderly alive much longer than in the past and worsening all the time. That is the downside of progress.

But if medical progress is a major driver of costs for the elderly, it is no less so for other age groups. *What Kind of Life: The Limits of Medical Progress* (1990) was meant to take a broader look at its impact on health care costs, but also to explore the status of medical progress as probably the most important ethical and social value underlying medical research and health care systems. An investment in science and a commitment to scientific progress was commonly invoked by America's founding fathers as vital for national welfare and human improvement. Progress in health care has rarely been examined in any critical way. Only with constant progress and the technological innovation that it generates, settled belief has held, can disease be eliminated or ameliorated and suffering reduced. And that has turned out to be true, and I am one of the beneficiaries of that progress. But I became drawn to the costs of that progress, economic and otherwise, and not just to its financial cost but also to our individual dignity of a wrecked body being kept alive by a medicine that, in its culture (if happily not always in its practice), has too little sense of when it should embrace, not fight, death.

Could the unconstrained pursuit of progress have the perverse effect of making health care increasingly unaffordable? My answer was yes, and our problem that of rethinking the meaning of progress and finding ways to pacify it. *What Kind of Life* got uniformly favorable notices, won me a book prize given by health care executives, and was reviewed enthusiastically on the first page of the *New York Times Book Review*. That was all any author could ask. But in the aftermath, I discovered that there was little taste for going after medical progress. The book and its thesis did not provoke, as I hoped it would, an interest in medical progress as a problem, not just a benefit. Progress continues to be treated as a self-evident good, immune from a critical examination. I gained praise for the book, but few followers for its thesis.

*The Troubled Dream of Life* had the aim in part of extending the examination of progress begun in *What Kind of Life*, but it mainly sought to remedy what I judged to be a great flaw in debates about end-of-life care. The flaw was its emphasis on patient choice, not on the substantive issue of the place of death in our lives. Care at the end of life was selected by us as one of the four main research topics that the Hastings Center would take on when it began. Complaints about that care had begun to emerge in the late 1960s, and it seemed an obvious candidate for examination. By the middle of the 1970s, and a series of conferences at the Center and elsewhere, a consensus seemed to emerge. It consisted of a three-part reform effort. The care of the dying would require choice on the part of patients about their treatment as they died, better education of physicians in the care of the dying, and improved palliative care and access to hospice care.

But a decade later, too little progress had been made with that reform plan. What was wrong? The most common explanation was a lack of strong implementation of the reform effort: too few people writing living wills or appointing a surrogate (no more than 20 percent in those days, and now 25 percent), continued poor training of physicians in the care of the dying, and persistent complaints about poor palliative care.

## The Missing Topic for End-of-Life Care: Death Itself

That was without doubt a plausible explanation, but I had come to think that effort had a serious omission. It did not include a professional, bioethical, or public discussion of death itself. Instead it had been turned into a legal, educational, and redefined medical problem (palliative care).

But how should we as individuals understand death in our own lives? How should medicine consider the place of death in the care of patients? The discussion bypassed those basic questions altogether.

What should we make of our universal fate, death? That is the kind of question that brings out what to me is a great weakness of liberal individualism: it has little place for, or tolerance of, public discussion of that kind of issue, bearing on what we make of life itself. The meaning of death had effectively been put off limits. The ordinary fear of death comes into play as well, creating its own obstacle to direct confrontation with its reality.

An argument with my editor at Simon & Schuster, the famous Alice Mayhew, about the title of the book forcefully brought the denial of death home to me. I wanted the title of the book to be *In Search of a Peaceful Death*. She firmly opposed that title: "We can't sell a book with the word 'death' in the title." I gave way, assuming she knew more about selling books than I did. Some six months later, Sherwin Nuland's book *How We Die* was published. It won the National Book Award and became a best-seller. Not long after that, the *New York Times* published a list of books on end-of-life care, all of which had "death" in the title. My book was not among them.

How could the compilers of that list have guessed from its title that my book was about death? The "troubled dream of life" was a phrase used by Montaigne, part of a sentence that said, "Death is a release from the troubled dream of life." I still like that sentence, but using just part of did not provide even a clue as to what the book was about. A few years later, when the paperback rights had been given to another publisher (Georgetown University Press), I was able to persuade the editor there (against some resistance once again) to use "In Search of a Peaceful Death" as the subtitle—what I wanted the original title to be.

The writing of three books over a decade, and the writing of many articles along the way, gave me renewed vitality at the Center, but possibly at a price. I had found that the only good antidote to my managerial fatigue was to create, with my writing, a separate life doing what gave me the greatest pleasure. The Center had gradually grown in size and budget over the first fifteen years, but I saw no reason for it to keep growing. We would not necessarily do better with a larger staff and I would not find an expanded administrative burden any benefit at all.

The status quo seemed perfectly good enough. Our capital campaign had been successful and a small endowment was in place. The hiring of a talented fundraiser, David K. Reeves, brought us considerable corporate support, almost all of it outside of the drug and device industries—which began to dry up by the late 1990s as corporate contribution policies began to change toward helping organizations more directly in their own interest.

I did not give much thought in those days to the future of the Center. From the beginning, Will and I saw the Center and the field as an adventure, not an effort to establish a permanent institution. Although during this period I should have been working harder to find some wealthy supporters to increase our endowment and strengthen annual giving, I was content enough chasing grants, which I always felt kept us helpfully nervous and creative, and I did not like at all the "cultivation" (that was the standard term) of the wealthy as a way of raising money. Fortunately, our current president, Tom Murray, has done a wonderful job in that respect and we have a much better, more helpful board of directors than we did during my term. I might have, if I had tried harder and put writing aside, left the Center in better shape when I retired in 1996.

### Straying from Bioethics: West Point, the U.S. Senate, and Higher Education

Apart from the lift that sustained writing gave me, there were a few events and projects that took us beyond the borders of bioethics into some unfamiliar territory: a project on the teaching of ethics in higher education, assisting West Point in establishing a program in ethics for the cadets, and a project to write a code of ethics for the U.S. Senate. All of those events took place for one reason: we had come to be looked upon as experts on ethics and its teaching by many of those outside of bioethics.

In 1980 I got a call from Colonel Peter Stromberg, chairman of the English Department at West Point. Stromberg, himself a graduate of the Academy and a Vietnam veteran, said that the Department of Defense had instructed the superintendent to establish an ethics program, and he had been assigned that task. The order for an ethics program was the result of a large-scale violation of the West Point honor code that led to the expulsion of more than a hundred cadets.

Peter's question to me was: how should we teach ethics? I said that we knew nothing about military ethics, and asked why he had come to us. He said he did not know where else he could get help and had heard of our work in medical ethics, so maybe we would have some ideas. That was an interesting challenge, and we set about trying to learn something about military ethics as well as passing along tips from our experience with the teaching of ethics in medical schools. Moreover, as a former army sergeant and high school cadet, I had an affection for the military. I learned how to live with blacks, poor whites, and all kinds of people whom I would not ordinarily encounter in my middle-class life, much less at Yale. This country would profit greatly from a required time for everyone to be in the military or some other kind of public service.

## Character Development and Ethical Analysis

An immediate difference appeared in the goal of teaching ethics in a military academy as compared with a medical school. In medical schools, the use of case studies was the standard practice, aiming to help the students to make difficult clinical decisions. The reigning tradition at West Point was the view that ethics teaching should aim to shape character. The point of the cadet honor code is to help instill and reinforce the West Point values of duty, honor, and country. We said that a common belief in bioethics teaching was that character could not be taught in a classroom, only an understanding of ethical rules, principles, and practices and their professional application.

I was probably more sympathetic to character development aspiration than many of my philosophy colleagues. But I was also wary of that as the emphasis, seeing how it had been trivialized by a common belief in medical schools that ethics teaching was nothing more than getting students to model themselves on the character and values of their senior teachers and clinical mentors. It had nothing to do with solving moral dilemmas or making good clinical judgments, taken to be a matter of scientific knowledge only.

We managed to persuade Colonel Stromberg and his colleagues that a combination of efforts were needed to get cadets to take seriously the kinds of values they should live by as military officers but also to grapple with ways to make good moral decisions not only on the battlefield but in ordinary military life as well. In any event, there have been no major failures of the honor code there in some thirty years that I have heard of, although I have been told it has been modified over the years, allowing more discretion in punishments and expulsion.

In 1997 the Hastings Center moved into a building in Garrison, New York, directly across the Hudson from West Point, making all the more convenient a thirty-year tradition of an annual meeting between the Academy's ethics faculty and the staff of the Center. A special event organized by West Point in 2009 to celebrate the Center's forteith anniversary was a particular treat, and the sword and scabbard presented to us on that occasion now graces the Center's hallway. We were also instrumental in the initiation of a national organization on military ethics, one that was at first for the three service academies but eventually became a worldwide organization for the military from many countries.

In 1980 we also organized a national conference on the teaching of ethics in higher education. As had happened with West Point, we began getting calls from teachers in a wide range of fields asking for our assistance with teaching ethics. Derek Bok, the president of Harvard, had written some influential articles on the need for ethics teaching, which in the earlier history of American higher education had an important role in the undergraduate curriculum. At the same time, a number of professional schools were introducing ethics courses. Derek's wife, philosopher Sissela Bok, was also interested and began collaborating with me to develop a collection of essays, *The Teaching of Ethics in Higher Education*.

Given all that activity, we organized a research project on the subject, culminating in a national conference. It was a great success, drawing representatives from ten professional fields and many teachers of undergraduate ethics. Despite the wide range of fields, each with different kinds of ethical problems to deal with and often very different teaching methods, all of the participants agreed that they shared a common pedagogical problem. They profited from hearing how others dealt with it: how to make the teaching of ethics interesting and pertinent to the personal lives and professional problems that their students would almost certainly encounter.

Those of us on the staff found especially interesting how many of those teaching professional ethics—whether in law, journalism, criminology, or business—found it hard to get their students to take the courses seriously. For all too many, regardless of the field, courses in ethics were taken to be a useless and boring distraction from the pursuit of professional skills. Hearing how the various teachers dealt with that problem was helpful. There seemed also to be a kind of informal competition among the conference participants about which kind of students were the most difficult to teach and which professions had the worst ethical problems. The easy winners (in the eyes of the Hastings staff) on difficult teaching were those who taught engineers, who were prone to little tolerance for something as fuzzy as ethics. They want straight answers, not provocative dilemmas.

The field of criminal justice won our prize for the worst ethical problems. From the policeman on the beat to the local prosecutor, daily discretionary decisions have to be made about whom to arrest or let off with a warning, or whom to prosecute and whose infraction of the law to overlook. The great difference between, say, a physician and someone in the criminal justice situation is that the latter have a lower social status. It is understood that doctors have to make wrenching decisions and that is a source of respect for them. Police officers are rarely lauded for making difficult arrest decisions.

### The Senate Code: Too Good to Be Plausible

Our assistance to the U.S. Senate came about much the same as it had with West Point. I got a call from the staff director of the Senate ethics committee. He and the chairman of the committee believed that they needed a formal and detailed code of ethics, which they did not have. Could we help them put one together? We said we knew nothing about legislative ethics, which was about as far from bioethics as military ethics. But I could not resist such a provocative invitation. I promptly accepted it and then, somewhat desperately, set out to find political scientists and others who could help. As it happened, we could locate no well-developed legislative codes at the state or local level, so everyone was more or less starting from scratch. We could hardly do worse than our predecessors, of which there were none.

We developed a conscientious and careful code, of which we felt the Senate could be proud. It paid solid attention to the bread-and-butter issues of financial probity and conflict of interest, but it also went well beyond that. We most wanted to paint a picture of an honest, thoughtful, and virtuous senator. Toward that end, we laid the heaviest burden on relationships with colleagues, conscientious committee service (attending meetings, reading necessary background reading, for instance), and in all things acting to enhance the public reputation of the Senate, which was rarely very high.

The code was presented at a hearing of the Select Committee on Ethics of the United State Senate on November 18, 1980. The committee chairman, Senator Howell Heflin, a Democrat from Alabama, praised us for it. Remarkably for a hearing, most of the committee members were present and stayed the whole time. Our effort was taken seriously. Each member of the Hastings team testified: Dan Clouser of the Penn State Medical School; Joel Fleishman from the Duke University School of Public Policy; Dennis Thompson, professor of politics at Harvard; and myself. We were carefully questioned and there were many lively interchanges.

What happened next? Nothing at all. The committee, we were told later by the staff director, decided to not use our code or any part of it. The reason was one we had not anticipated. The committee decided that our kind of code was just inappropriate for a political body. Although it was important to have ethical rules and regulations pertaining to money and conflict of interest, that was as far as it should go. Whether senators were conscientious in fulfilling their duties, respectful of colleagues, and hard-working committee members was a matter for the voters to decide. It was their standards and judgments, not those of the Senate itself, that were to count.

There wasn't anything wrong per se with our proposed standards of conduct. But they were, the message seemed to be, more appropriate for a Boy Scout troop than for elected public officials. Whether those reasons were a way of evading a serious ethical code, or politics as usual, or simply a reasonable political point, we could not judge. But as would become more fully obvious later when I began to work on the 2008–2009 health reform effort, ethics as understood in the political arena is different from that discussed in the classroom and academic journals. It is not just that one is serious and the other cynical, or that one rational and the other emotional. The mix is different. Our work with the Senate was a good foretaste.

## Ethics and Emotions

In 1980 my wife Sidney received her Ph.D. in social psychology. That led her to write a book on the role of emotions in ethics, *In Good Conscience: The Role of Reason and Emotion in Moral Decision Making*. That topic was chosen for a fortuitous combination of motives. One of them was that psychology was just discovering the emotions and their relationship to reason and cognitive judgments. The other was that she had been surprised at many of the Hastings Center meetings by the hostility to emotion expressed by most of the philosophers. Emotions were seen as the enemy of reason, something to be banished in order to think clearly. Roderick Firth's ideal observer (chapter 1) was the prototype: detached, objective, rational and all-seeing. But the psychological research was discovering that reason and emotion are intertwined.

Every reason has an emotional component, and every emotion has a cognitive component. In later years, my friend and early colleague Leon R. Kass provoked not just disagreement but outright personal hostility for commending the "wisdom of repugnance" as a guide to ethics. "Wisdom" was too strong a word because, as even he acknowledged, our emotions, including repugnance, can turn out to be wrong. Some obvious instances are the repugnance felt by many at people of a different race or the concept that women should be able to vote. Yet I also had to recall the other side of the repugnance coin, rarely mentioned: repugnance as an early sense that something was wrong but for which there was available no rational justification. As a teenager in Washington, D.C., I felt a repugnance at the way African Americans were treated, but I had no social or intellectual support for that emotion in a segregated, heavily southern, city; the early American abolitionists were in a similarly weak position. It just turned out that our repugnance was correct.

As a result of Sidney's work, I became interested in the role of emotion in decision making but also that of world views and ideological influences on clinical and policy decisions. My own research and writing on rationing, limits, and progress required crossing back and forth over the unclear boundary line between ethics and politics. Why was there so much disagreement on some issues (abortion) yet so little on others (informed consent for medical research)? Reasons—and repugnances—that seemed flatly wrong to some seemed self-evident to others. The differences were not of the same kind that had historically troubled philosophers about the incompatibility of competing ethical theories. I call the differences "ideological" because they seem to embody a combination of theoretical differences and conflicting emotions, both mixed with cultural influences that push people in one direction or another. It is as if the culture provides the emotions and passions and the ideologies the rationale for accepting them. It is not necessarily, as David Hume averred, that "reason is the slave of the passions" (although it surely can be) but that the passions are made sense of by the culture of different communities. Reason and emotion work in tandem, not as slaves and masters.

Attitudes toward the rationing of health care for the elderly seem to me particularly interesting. They represent an instance in which two distinct ideologies are used to accept what recent culture has succeeded in inculcating in us, that of giving the elderly the same equality for the allocation of resources as every other age group. From the left, the resistance to rationing is a function of liberal individualism in the Enlightenment mode: every age group has a full and equal right to the benefits of medical progress, and it is the obligation of government to insure that equality.

From the right, resistance to rationing by government, as would be the case in the Medicare program, is based on the market presumption that everyone should have the market freedom to choose the care they want at all ages. The right is particularly opposed to rationing by government, as would be the case in the Medicare program. Despite a belief in deficit reduction and downsizing of government, they have, inconsistently, often opposed any benefit reduction in Medicare. The combination of the voting power of the elderly, not to be ignored, and an acceptance of equality among the different age groups has put them in an untenable ideological position. The future course of the reform implementation will see how that contradiction is resolved. The Democrats have no less of a problem. Holding onto the aim of keeping the number of uninsured low and finding a point of solvency for Medicare will entail rationing—cutting desired or even efficacious benefits. Rationality will have to overcome ideology for a sustainable health care system.

## Stepping Down

By 1995 I had decided that the time was coming for me to step down as director of the Hastings Center, which I did in 1996. I had accomplished all that I set out to do, the Center was financially stable, and it was time to let go. The language I used in writing my own announcement was to describe the change in status as that of "stepping down," not "retiring." I was not old enough in my self-estimation to retire! But I discovered that if one steps down from a position at 45, the assumption is that one will move on to a new job—not so at 66. Whatever I wanted to call it, everyone else called it "retiring." They knew, as I knew, that I had no interest in a new job, nor was anyone offering me one.

I was simply doing what more and more older people were doing: scaling back on work time, doing only what they wanted to do (if they could get away with it), and most of all shedding day-to-day management responsibilities.

Interested in that phenomenon, I did some research and calculated that for most people in white-collar occupations, forty years or so was the limit of their tolerance for full-time work with significant responsibilities. I had worked as an administrator just under forty years. The relevance of that observation is that, if I'm more or less correct, the expectation that more and more people will want to work full time beyond age 65 doing what they always did is unlikely; a part-time retirement will be more attractive. And if forced to continue working by lack of adequate retirement resources, not all will be happy, particularly as they move into their 80s. I have been one of the lucky ones, continuing to enjoy my work and especially blessed by my interest is a set of issues (such as health care reform) that have taken center stage of late. Of course, if the elderly stay in the workforce at high levels in future years, as the current recession is forcing many to do, they will block the entry of the young, creating a new and unpleasant moral and social dilemma—just the kind that would preoccupy me in my post–"stepping down" years.

# 6
## Opening the Floodgates: 1996–2010

When I stepped down from the Hastings Center in 1996, I had no clear agenda or any particular ambitions. I knew I would write, always had and always will, but I had no immediate topics in mind. I was given a six-month sabbatical by the Center and, through the good offices of Sissela Bok, spent that time at the Harvard Center for Population and Development Studies on Bow Street, just off Harvard Square. That was a most congenial appointment, taking me back to my 1969 work on population policy and reawakening the memories of my graduate days at Harvard, mainly the pleasant ones.

Just to remind me that age was creeping up, I began having breathing problems that year. I was diagnosed as an asthmatic, which was then added to an earlier diagnosis of moderate emphysema. I was not one of those persons who said, "Why me?" It seemed only fair that I begin experiencing the problems of aging and illness about which I had been copiously writing. Perhaps curiously, as I began accumulating assorted ailments and accompanying hospital time, nothing I actually experienced changed my thinking but merely confirmed what I had earlier gathered from reading and observation. We will see what the next few years will bring in that respect. I can't wait. No, that's wrong. Yes, I can. Will I have a choice? No.

As it turned out, these later years have been among the most productive of my career, mainly because of my writing but no less because of various other activities as well. My thinking about ethics advanced, in great part because I took up issues that were outside of mainstream bioethics, requiring research in wholly new areas. I have often been asked what has been most important for my own pleasure and satisfaction, my writing or my role in starting and running the Center. I have little doubt that the life span of the Center will outlive my books, but I am much more attached to my writing. The main difference between being a writer and an administrator is that my computer does not talk back to me or throw up emotional tangles of the kind that managing people does—and I don't have to raise money to use it.

I did one thing during those years I had rarely done before and thought I never would again: teaching. Flying up to Boston once a week, I taught a seminar on ethics and health policy at the Harvard Medical School from 1998 to 2006. It was an irresistible assignment, about as ideal as one could ask and overcoming my aversion to teaching. It had an average of three students a semester. They were mainly in their late 20s and early 30s, invariably had degrees in law or some other professional field, and regardless of what I had assigned, had already read about half of it. I had little to do other than moderate their discussions with each other, sprinkling bits of elder wisdom about.

Hardly less predictable earlier was an effort I undertook in 2007 to establish a relationship between Yale and the Hastings Center. I had at the time an appointment (no pay and no clear duties) as a Senior Scholar at Yale and began musing about some kind of affiliation. I had not developed a late-in-life romance with universities—far from it—but I felt that the staff at the Center would benefit from a collaboration, which I likened to a "relationship" in the contemporary sense of that term, not a marriage. In 2009 the Yale-Hastings Program in Ethics in Health Policy was established. It took two years to move through the Yale bureaucracy—notable, I was told, for its sluggishness—reminding me often why we chose not to be at a university. So far it has gone well.

## The Outbreak of the Culture Wars

An important event for me in those years was dealing with the culture wars that had broken out in the field. Up until the early 2000s, bioethics was, as described earlier, mainly in the hands of liberals, many of them resistant to religion and conservative ideas. That began to change, as more conservatives were drawn to the field—but most often it seemed as critics of the field itself. That was fueled in part by the Reagan and Bush years and the neoconservatism that went with it. Journals such as *First Things*, the *National Review*, and the *Weekly Standard* began publishing broadside attacks on bioethics, often designating Peter Singer as our appointed leader (he wasn't) but mainly identifying the field as one marked by just the kind of liberalism, ethical relativism, and moral decay that needed curbing.

An important figure in that camp was Leon R. Kass, from the American Enterprise Institute and the University of Chicago. He had been one of the first recruits when we founded the Center, served on our board for years, and took part in many research projects. He was also a good friend and someone whose writings I much admired. As time had gone on, however, he turned on the field, joining the conservative critics. As was characteristic of many of those critics, he rarely singled out any liberal person or position to argue against. It was a broad critique that did not acknowledge the diversity of opinions, by no means all of it liberal. It was also marked by an unpleasant kind of self-serving rhetoric, with frequent phrases such as "right-thinking" and "thoughtful" and "serious" people who shared conservative views. I came to think of most conservatives as ethically serious but often not intellectually rigorous, at least in the sense of carefully argued, well-footnoted, academic-style publications. That essay style of writing was well polished by Irving Kristol, a neoconservative leader who mainly wrote that way. It is also a style well adapted to leading a movement.

There was an assumption, it seems to me, that the solution to most bioethical problems could be found in the Western great books, classical literature, and religious traditions. But the classics appeared to be invoked for their rhetorical power rather than as the basis for carefully formulated arguments. Gravitas was worn heavily on their rhetorical sleeve. They did not find it necessary to engage in conventional direct intellectual arguments with liberals, responding with a careful critique of their views and naming names: the criticisms tend to be generic and sweeping. Most disturbing has been their failure to come to grips with the devastating impact of market values on our society (which Kristol had acknowledged). Market ideas and practices are a solvent of all traditions, relativistic to the extreme, destructive of moral values—and pervasive in American medicine and biomedical research. To what extent there is a self-censorship induced by the support many conservatives have from business-supported foundations and think tanks is something I wonder if they think about.

## Meeting with the President and Karl Rove

In the summer of 2001 I received a call from Karl Rove asking me if I would meet with President George W. Bush to discuss stem cell research. Kass had been invited and suggested me as someone who would have a judgment different from his. For reasons I could never understand, he thought I would be a supporter of the research. That was not the case, as anyone else who knew me would have realized. In fact, there were some who saw it all as a kind of conspiracy, with Leon smuggling in another opponent to the research under the pretext that I would have a different view. All the more oddly, Leon seemed to me during the meeting to be ambivalent, while I was firmly opposed. (I will explain my stance more fully shortly.) As for the meeting with the president, it turned out that he and his advisors were mainly considering the policy they eventually chose: that of allowing research with spare embryos created before a specific date. I had not given much thought to that possibility, about which I did not have much to say.

I was frequently asked later what the meeting was like. Not particularly interesting, I said, mainly because the president, Karl Rove, and Karen Hughes simply threw questions at us, rarely responding to our answers or opening an exchange. The meeting lasted an hour and a half, which I was told later was remarkably long for the president. I petted his Scotch terrier and said I had seen President Roosevelt's similar dog, Fala, while growing up in Washington. I am generally more favorable to Scotch terriers than Republican presidents. President Bush was surprised when I said I was pro-choice on abortion, but then so are most people, because it's an uncommon combination. Leroy Walters from Georgetown also met with the president, but we have never had a chance to compare our experiences.

A few months later, Leon was appointed chairman of the newly formed President's Council on Bioethics. The general composition of the council was weighted toward conservatives but was by no means monolithic in its composition or reports. Most disturbing for me was the hostility, and often outright nastiness, directed at Kass and the council by many bioethicists and some writers in the media. The council did solid work and Kass was a hard-working and conscientious director. Did I agree with everything he said? No, but then what of it? Disagreements have been a mark of bioethics since the beginning. He was being tarred in part because of his association and George W. Bush, with little attention paid to the reports of his council.

## The Attack on Kass: An Embarrassment for the Field

Kass did not deserve those attacks. I was acutely embarrassed that people in my field were behaving with exactly the kind of meanness and political partisanship that was becoming so destructive of civilized political discourse. Hardly any of the critics seemed to notice that every other presidential commission had, with minor exceptions, been uniformly liberal, in staff and commission members. No one had complained about that. The last thing a field that professed to be serious about ethics needed was a culture war. It made us look foolish. I later organized a conference at the Center to bring liberals and conservatives in together and then followed up with a series of small meetings. I was distressed afterwards that two prominent conservatives, Yuval Levin and Eric Cohen, who had worked with Kass and who had been to my meetings, published an article in 2010 attacking President Obama's new bioethics commission, the Presidential Commission for the Study of Bioethical Issues, before it had even issued one word, and promised to shadow its predictably bad stuff. Its tone and invective were exactly those of Kass's liberal critics. But Kass, I later discovered, had made a slightly disparaging remark about the policy emphasis of earlier commissions.

## The Goals of Medicine and Sustainable Health Care

At the time of my retirement in 1996, the Center published a report on a project I had organized, *The Goals of Medicine: Setting New Priorities.* My aim was to determine whether medical progress, the increase of chronic illness, and rising costs required a revision of the traditional goals of medicine. The project was international, with fourteen countries represented. It was later translated into six other languages and led to a series of conferences in other countries. But it did not gain much attention here, and perhaps we needed such a discussion most of all. Although the other countries represented in the project were having trouble with the costs and quality of their health care systems, none were in as bad shape as the United States, few were as addicted to progress as the United States, and medical paternalism was still the rule.

Once again I saw how idiosyncratic our health system is. I envied the universal care of the other countries, but that feature did not seem transferable, and they felt there was little to learn from us. The failure of the Clinton reform effort in 1993 suggested that the United States had a long way to go before there would be any significant change. Yet the mid-90s would be remembered for one historically unique feature: the success of health maintenance organizations (HMOs) in holding down annual cost increases. That was a short-lived triumph, killed by a combination of physician and patient complaints. Neither group was willing to tolerate a strong, central role for government. I later decided that the *Goals of Medicine* report had been too bland and too vague about what new priorities were needed. But I had not given up on the problem, remaining convinced that sooner or later the conventional, settled goals would have to be changed.

My 1998 book *False Hopes: Why America's Quest for Perfect Health Is a Recipe for Failure* was an attempt to make a stronger case and with more detail. But if lightning does not strike twice in the same place, that does not mean one can't be a sucker twice in the same way. The same editor who did not like the word "death" in a book on death objected to the title I wanted for the book. What I had in mind was "sustainable medicine," bringing into health care a common term in the environmental movement. I aimed to lay out was a vision for the future of medicine and health that was economically sustainable in the long run, equitably available and commanding popular support. That will mean a steady-state for health care costs, leveling off at an affordable level, with annual costs limited to the annual growth of general costs, in the range of 3 percent a year.

My editor refused to accept the word "sustainable," saying that it was just a technical jargon term that no one would understand. We compromised on *False Hopes*, which did not catch my thesis at all and was to boot positively misleading and baffling to at least a few reviewers. Just to make certain I never forget how dumb I was to give in on the title, the phrase "sustainable health care" is now a common one, but rarely connected with anything I wrote. There was a bit of solace in the use of the phrase (and was attributed to me) in Canadian health care policy, but Canadians were not the audience I was aiming for. Live and don't learn.

But writing *False Hopes* got me hooked on health care reform, a topic of interest to only a few in bioethics but much larger in American politics and health policy. Out of my work in Eastern Europe, I became interested in health care systems there and in other European countries as well. I had long admired those latter systems, particularly their universal care and much lower costs, but was surprised that all of them—regardless of the many differences in their organization—were having problems holding down costs. They did better than the United States, but they were also talking about an "unsustainable" growth in costs.

## Medicine and the Market

Of special interest to me was their common flirtation with and sometimes a real marriage to otherwise scorned market values and practices, often invoking—of all places—the United States as a model (and particularly our HMOs). I first noticed this during my trips to the Czech Republic and the Netherlands. No sooner had the Velvet Revolution taken place in the former country, the new government transformed its health care system with many market strategies and considerable privatization of many government institutions. The Netherlands did not go so far but had invited Alain Enthoven, a conservative economist and supporter of managed care, to help them bring more market practices and policies into its system. The Czech experience was a disaster that drove costs up, not down, and was mainly abandoned after a few years. Not so with the Netherlands, which continued down a market path and in 2006 instituted a radical reform in a market direction. It has not worked well there either.

*Medicine and the Market: Equity v. Choice* (1996) was my response to those observations. I was curious about the market and its future in our country but also what inroads it was making in developed and developing countries. I recruited a colleague at the Center, Angela Wasunna, a native of Kenya and a lawyer, to coauthor the book with me. We divided up the writing of the book. I would examine the developed countries and she would examine the developing countries. I knew it would be necessary to read about the history of market thinking and the voluminous work of health care economist on health care and the market.

Economists, I was told as I started out, tended to be favorable toward the market, but from an efficiency and not an ethical perspective, and I found that generally to be true. But beyond the work of economists, I soon became interested in the power of market ideology in the United States and the great debate that ideology played in the run-up to the reform efforts that were brewing. I became a zealous reader of the *Wall Street Journal* and *Forbes,* periodically dipping into the *Weekly Standard* and the *National Review.* I still have a large collection of books by proselytizing market proponents, a high percentage of whose authors taught in business schools. The market was treated as a moral, not just an efficiency value. At its heart is a belief, almost religious in its intensity, that individual consumer choice and (mainly) unfettered competition among providers is the key to a good heath care system.

## The Failure of Competition

The power of the market through competition, they hold, works brilliantly to bring down the price of consumer goods including automobiles, TVs, and cell phones, and can just as surely do it with health care services. Moreover, as an added bonus, the health and vitality of the market are critical for the vitality and strength of democracy. But I came away from my immersion in market zeal and literature with a problem. It seems to an act of compelling faith. I could find no strong evidence anywhere that market practices work to hold down health care costs, whatever their value for purchasers of TV screens or cell phones. As the available evidence showed, competition mainly pushes costs up. Private insurance premiums regularly rise every year, faster than the annual cost of living. American hospitals regularly compete with each other for patients by touting the latest and best technologies—at higher and higher costs. The common market proponent response was that government regulation of health care stifled competition; get the government off our backs and economic miracles in health care will blossom. It was hard to find evidence for that belief.

Most striking was the absence of any apparent concern for the uninsured or the victims of market failure. The market sensibility showed, to me at least, that the market individualism that stood behind it—the identical twin of the individualism of political liberalism—was little interested in ideas of the common good. The latter was, if you will, my ideology. I was drawn to the European value of solidarity, which has always seemed to me a more potent value for health care than the language of rights or justice. I understand solidarity to represent a recognition of our finitude, our common vulnerability to illness and suffering, and our dependence upon others to reduce and ameliorate that vulnerability. We are, in short, all in this together, sharing the same fate.

Solidarity depends on our empathy for others. Arguments for a right to health care, or a justice claim, do not require that or ordinarily try to evoke it. The most effective case for universal health care draws upon the stories and images of the sad state of those without insurance. That was the power of Michael Moore's documentary *Sicko*. One ultimately has to be able to feel and understand the pain of others, mainly strangers, to willingly be taxed to help them, It was impossible for market proponents to show how choice and competition is of any use at all to those who lack the money to choose anything. It is no less implausible to use concepts of rights to do the work of empathy, and far harder with so-called positive rights (our claim on something from our neighbor) than negative rights (our claim to be left alone to live our life as we choose).

If I had even once in the reform debate heard a market proponent say that he recognized that the freedom sought in the market could inadvertently do harm to others, that it did at least pose a dilemma in the face of suffering, I might have had greater respect for the market argument. But it was as if the uninsured did not even exist, or, more precisely, as if there were a strong conservative effort to minimize their number, to whittle away the standard government number of 45,000. When that effort could not succeed, there was always the backup contention that because the uninsured could always get free emergency care, there was little reason for nanny government, European welfare state–style, to intervene. Emergency care, however, does not get one into the rest of the hospital, where the really large costs are.

## The Oregon Rationing Plan

*Medicine and the Market* was my first foray into ordinary health policy, even though my writing on sustainability and limits to health care touched on some important features of it. I eventually wrote one more book on health policy, *Taming the Beloved Beast* (2009), but in the meantime I took a detour. In the late 1980s I had a small hand in assisting Dr. John Kitzhaber, then Director of Health in Oregon and later to become its governor, in formulating his plan for a priority system for allocating treatments in the state's Medicaid program. In the end, some 700 conditions were prioritized. There were many liberal critics of the program, mainly because it was seen as in effect a rationing system, which was true, but one that unfairly picked upon the poor, which was not true. The state had to take on the costs of the Medicaid program and decided upon the priority plan as the best way to do that. Dr. Kitzhaber told me later that I was the only philosopher who had been helpful to him.

Kitzhaber's strategy recognized a point often noted about universal care systems in different parts of the world: most of them have annual budgets, which are unavoidable and which force the setting of priorities. Medicaid in Oregon was government financed by a combination of federal and state money, and it had an annual budget. That budget had to be rationed, and the most obvious way to do it was to prioritize available care from the most necessary and urgent to the least necessary. During the same period, a number of European countries such as Denmark and the Netherlands were pursuing prioritization strategies as well, and an international organization of priorities in health care was established.

## Priority Setting in Research

Yet there was a surprising omission in the priority movement. Why was there no discussion about setting priorities in biomedical research, but only in health care delivery? I decided to take that question on. As it happened, also in the late 1990s, Congress requested that the Institute of Medicine (IOM) create a group to study how the NIH set its research priorities. Of all the federal agencies, the NIH was probably the most blessed. Its annual budget showed a steady, unbroken rise since World War II, by then close to $30 billion a year, an almost perfect record of bipartisan support, and a public over the years wholeheartedly supportive of a strong government role in research. When Congress asked for an IOM study, it was mainly because a few voices were beginning to push NIH to show that it was doing a good job spending well the money appropriated for it. The IOM Commission, directed by Leon Rosenberg, a former dean of the Yale Medical School, determined that its priority-setting strategies—some six criteria—were adequate but did not in the end state how they were to be ranked or what the procedure was to say how that was to be done. A real prioritization system would have to find a way to do just that.

I was disappointed that hardly anyone followed up with further studies of priority setting in research, and nothing much seems to have come from it at the NIH. But I remained interested in the topic, particularly recalling it in 1998 when James Thomson of the University of Wisconsin announced his research on the potential medical benefits of embryonic stem cell research. And then, under another layer of memory, I recalled that the NIH in the mid-1990s had convened a panel on the use of embryos for research. When I went back to that study, entirely favorable to such research, I noted a peculiarity of the way it laid out its thinking. The issue was presented as one that required a balancing of two important values: the moral status of embryos against the lives that might be saved by using them for clinical and research purposes.

Yet the report devoted two chapters to the embryo problem, deciding that they could be used, but not a single sentence defending the moral rationale for research, as if that were too self-evident to even assess—and thus automatically giving research the highest priority. I then recalled Paul Ramsey's phrase in the 1970s from the debate on the use of children for research purposes, criticizing Richard McCormick defense of that practice as dependent on an implicit "research imperative," a moral obligation to carry out any research that might have a health benefit. Nor could I forget Hans Jonas's contention that medical research is melioristic, which is a human good but is not a moral obligation. I then decided to write a book on the idea of a research imperative.

## The Research Imperative: A Human Good, Not an Obligation

That book, *What Price Better Health: Hazards of the Research Imperative* (2003), had two purposes. One of them was to combat the idea that there is a research imperative for medical research—a moral obligation to pursue it—and the other was to fill out the idea of "research ethics" (to encompass a wide range of ethical issues in research, not just human subject research), a term that hitherto had been limited to the ethics of human subject research. I resist the idea of a research imperative for three reasons. First, if it did not include some way to set priorities (better than the current NIH method), there will be no way to counteract a particularly discouraging reality about medical research: it is a main engine for rising costs. A general correlation between research expenditures and costs has been noted for many years by health care economists, with little dissent. That is not to deny that some research has and will reduce costs, just not most research. The likely reason is that research has led to a variety of successful but increasingly expensive ways to prolong the lives of sick people, most notably those of the chronically ill. Cures have been few and far between for decades now.

A second reason to resist research as if it is a self-evident good is that little if any interest has been paid in our society to its opportunity costs, as economists would put it, that of alternative and perhaps better ways of spending the money. The socioeconomic determinants of health are by now well known, particularly education, income, and a healthy social environment. It is hard to think of any serious public discussion of spending less on health care and more on education and job creation. It was hardly noted in the debate, moreover, that the NIH was already spending billions each year for research on the very diseases that stem cell research was to conquer in the years ahead.

A third reason is that the present de facto priority given to lethal disease (primarily diseases of the elderly)—the NIH leaders in research spending for decades have been cancer, heart disease, and stroke—takes away money for less lethal conditions and those, such as mental health, that do not kill but make life a misery. The warfare against the diseases of aging is a losing battle, never to be won but capable of consuming large amounts of money. The death of people in old age has never been considered in any society some kind of national tragedy. But we seem to have turned it into that by giving it the highest health care research priority. Better priorities could be set, centering on quality of life rather than length of life. As an addendum, I would add, I did not believe that my support for freedom of choice in abortion and thus a killing of embryos (and fetuses) in any way entailed using them for research purposes. Embryos have a weak moral claim but the claim of medical research is even weaker.

Some thirteen years after Thompson's research on embryonic stem cells, there have been no significant clinical developments, much less cures. The emphasis now is on its value for research. Meanwhile, adult stem cell research, earlier often haughtily dismissed as inferior in promise, has steadily advanced in its medical uses. But then, we might recall, the Human Genome Project, mapping the human genome, has not led to any medical cures despite its "promise" (the term of money-raising art) of getting to the genetic bottom of all human disease. And this is some nine years after the publication of *What Price Better Health*, I add ruefully, which was a book that had little impact in bioethics, neither the book itself nor its effort to look more fully and closely at medical research. But then, like human genome and embryonic research, my assessment of research itself may yet bear fruit. Maybe tomorrow, or maybe some day, or just maybe. As a reader of murder mysteries, I have learned that the settled police wisdom is that if murders are not solved quickly, they are likely never to be solved. Is something like that true with highly touted, promising scientific breakthroughs and books?

## Technology and Health Care Costs

I wrote *Taming the Beloved Beast: How Medical Technology Costs Are Destroying Our Health Care System* (2009) just as the health reform debate was heating up, and it was published at the moment in the fall of 2009 when the final legislation was all but assured. Technology had been, for my entire career in bioethics, the thread connecting almost all of the ethical problems I worked on. It was technological developments (organ transplantation) that forced the brain definition of death, the first Hastings Center project in 1970. It was the advent of prenatal diagnosis around the same time that forced some new childbearing decisions on parents. It was medicine's steadily enhanced power to keep dying patients alive with new technologies that created the dilemmas marking end-of-life care. It was the prospect of genetic engineering that excited and alarmed both scientists and the public. Looking back, it is hard to think of any major issue we took on that did not have new technologies as their genesis.

I think I have always been ambivalent about science and technology, and perhaps that is where my Catholic background reveals itself. I had three years of science at my Catholic military school, biology, chemistry, and physics. But it was taught as something an educated person should know about, important but not something that most of us would have much to do with as citizens or professionally. Only one of my fellow students, out of a class of a hundred, went into science, at MIT. Chastened by its treatment of Galileo, the church had long before accepted science, including evolution.

It was only in comparison with Jews and Protestants that a difference in intensity was obvious. C. P. Snow once wrote, in his *Two Cultures*, that scientists have "the future in their bones." I doubt that many Catholics shared that expectation. There was among Jews, especially those who had moved in a secular direction, an enthusiasm about science, a belief in it far more intense than among Catholics. My wife's Protestant background led her to believe that when she had grown up, medicine would have cured most diseases, possibly even death itself. The number of Catholic Nobel laureates is miniscule in comparison with Protestants and Jews. And of course there has always been a strong correlation between nonreligious secularists and a faith in science as the royal road to truth. In college, failing my biology course, I quickly gravitated toward the humanities, choosing one side of the two cultures for cultivation and not the other.

## The Seductive Myths of Technology

Yet although I was an outsider to science, looking on at it but not caught up in it with the fervor common to most Americans, I was nonetheless fascinated by the way science and technology were, like it or not, shaping our culture, our lives, and the human future. I could hardly deny the benefits of technology, medical and otherwise, in my own life and that of others. But the dropping of the atom bombs on Hiroshima and Nagasaki was, even for a 15-year-old, enough evidence for a lifetime that technology was the greatest of all two-edged swords. I rejected early on the two most common myths about technology. One of them is that technology is a neutral power, entirely dependent upon how we use it. As the gun lobby says, guns don't kill—only people do. But the very presence of technology in our lives does change the way we behave. It is thus utterly predictable that if you flood a neighborhood or town with hand guns, the murder and accident rate from gun deaths will go up.

The second and related myth is that technology merely expands the range of choices in our life, which we can take or leave as we see fit. But it is hard for a pregnant woman to turn down amniocentesis, now a standard part of obstetrical care. And it's even harder to turn down the use of a telephone, first the old-fashioned land-line kind and now the cell phone. Some New Yorkers manage to live without automobiles, but that is just about impossible for the rest of us. In many instances, it is the market in action that seductively grabs us by the hand and pulls us along. But we are the ones who hold out our hands to make that possible. As I write this, the news is full of stories about "promising" breakthroughs in the early diagnosis of Alzheimer's disease. My own view is that it would be foolishness squared to take such a test, with no serious prospect of a cure or forestalling of its symptoms much later in the offing. But I have no doubt that there will be many people who will want it.

### Taming the Beloved Beast

All of this has been a long introduction to what I want to say about my book *Taming the Beloved Beast*. Writing that book brought out, from some depths or other, years of musing about ethics and technology, and no less what I came to think of as a deep and troubling moral dilemma. Put in its simplest terms, the dilemma is that the high and ever-growing cost of medical technology can bring a health care system to financial ruin and can jeopardize the life and health of almost everyone in it.

The peculiarly troublesome part of the dilemma is that it is hard to deny or even minimize its health benefits, and no less hard to deny the financial and other benefits from the lives it can save. Patients want it, doctors are trained and well paid to prescribe and use it, and the drug and device industries make billion selling it. Along the way it provides hundreds of thousands of jobs. But it is also the main reason for ever-rising health care costs (some 50 percent of annual cost escalation), which plague not only our health care system but every other one as well. It is a beloved beast because it gives us health and pleasure, saving our lives and relieving our suffering, but is also almost uncontrollable in its economic fallout. It is a beast that so far has resisted training, at least in the United States. I think my basic point is a simple one, and with a solid empirical basis, but many people seem to have fixed in their minds such a positive view of technology that they cannot imagine how it could, at the same time, be a threat. But that combination is just the way it has turned out.

The main strategy in other developed countries to control costs is strong government controls on the supply and price of technologies. The price of drugs and devices is regulated, care is taken in the way they are disseminated, and physicians have few financial incentives to use them. There are some important cultural restraints as well. Public opinion polls indicate less desire for expensive technologies than in our country. The media does not report as extensively on medical research or with the often breathless excitement of the U.S. media. And everywhere there are (with some exceptions) fewer heart procedures, dialysis units, surgical procedures, and less costly drugs. Even so, the European countries get better health outcomes at lower cost and with greater patient satisfaction. But one does not have to spend much time in Europe, where annual cost escalation is in the 3 to 5 percent range, to find pervasive anxiety about the financial sustainability of their systems. They are faced with the same underlying dynamic as we are: rapidly aging populations and an accompanying steady rise in chronic disease, high expectations about the quality of care, and a steady stream of new and improved technologies.

## The Timeless Failure to Control Costs

The United States has had little success over the decades in controlling costs, an effort that began with the Nixon administration in 1970. The annual cost escalation has fluctuated between 6 and 10 percent, and most recently settled in around 6 percent—a rate capable of doubling overall health care costs in a decade or so. Only for a few years in the mid-1990s did the escalation cease, and then not for long in the face of opposition to the successful HMO efforts to rein in costs. Most of the efforts to control costs assume that the main villains are waste and inefficiency, abetted by a fee-for-service medicine that provides financial incentives for physicians to use technology.

Intense merchandising efforts by the medical industrial community to sell its products to physicians and direct-to-consumer advertising to reach consumers no doubt contribute to waste and the overuse of drugs and devices. But none of the essentially managerial efforts have worked with any effectiveness: almost everything in American culture and that of American medicine favors technology and almost everything (aided by conservative resistance) works against its control. Cures have been few and far between for decades now. The 2009 health reform legislation put in many measures that could bring about a great change (which I will not go into here). It will take at least a full decade for them to take effect, with many obstacles along the way. Like everyone else, I await the implementation of the legislation with uncertainty and trepidation. Medical technology has been the golden calf of modern American medicine, but a Moses has yet to appear to overthrow it.

### Editing a Blog on Cost Control

Although *Taming the Beloved Beast* was published just as the health reform effort was successfully winding down, the book had been finished some eighteen months earlier (academic publishers are slow), and some of it was already a little outdated. I wanted the book to play some role, however small, in the debate, but it came out a few months too late to make that possible. Looking for an alternative way of staying in the fray, I persuaded my colleagues at the Center to let me start a blog on cost control, which seemed increasingly marginalized in the final months of the debate.

My colleagues found the idea of a blog a good one but were surprised that I was the one who thought of it. I was not known as someone who read blogs, and actually I never did before or after I started my own. But I had learned through the old-fashioned, now declining, print media that millions of Americans did. And there were at least fifty blogs on health care out there already. My own experience in writing on age and rationing for the *New York Times* had generated a large overnight response, and I was impressed. Unlike most blogs, mine was to be edited by me and a colleague, Susan Gilbert, with a variety of contributors (of which I was one, many times).

The blog (http://www.healthcarecostmonitor.org) got hundreds of "hits," as the jargon had it; we personally received many nice comments about it; and it was rated one of the best health policy blogs. But did it make any difference? There was no way of telling, but it did not appear that way. I posted entries by many important figures in health policy: Henry Aaron, Alain Enthoven, Jacob Hacker, Richard Saltman, and Louise Russell, as well as Norman Daniels, Peter Ubel, and Leonard Fleck from bioethics. But it became evident as the debate on costs moved along that academic and other health policy experts were far overshadowed by partisan politics and special interests (both ideological and financial).

I wrote an article some months later for the *Hastings Center Report*, following up on blogs we had published on rationing. I noted how no one at all of any consequence politically had used that word in the reform debate, and how Republicans, despite their repeated avowal of the need for cost cutting, were the first to label any tough steps as rationing, one of the most effective killer words politically. The gap between the careful language of academic and think tank analysts—almost too careful, with its analytic coolness—and that of the political operatives, with few emotional restraints, came to seem huge and unbridgeable. John Rawls got huge play in the academy, but none of consequence outside of it, just as rationing got careful attention in the professional journals but was either bypassed altogether in congressional discussions or used as an ideological curse word. I was an editor of a blog, but not a dedicated reader of that medium; I was nonetheless both impressed by the importance of the social media and a politicization of old-school TV and radio. In health policy, moreover—a highly specialized field—it was the journal article or the downloadable foundation or think tank report was the communication medium of choice.

After my 1998 book, *False Hopes*, was published by Simon & Schuster, my editor (the one who did not like the words "death" or "sustainability") informed me that they would not publish any more of my books. *False Hopes* had sold only 5,000 copies in the first year, no longer a decent number in a trade book industry marked by a steady decline in book sales and an attempt to compensate by looking for blockbusters. I hope my friends at my four subsequent academic publishers—the University of California Press, Johns Hopkins, MIT, and Princeton—will not mind my saying so, but I felt demoted to second string. It was hard to give up fast-track trade book publishing schedules (eight or nine months), paid book tours, a blessed freedom from peer review, a generous advertising budget, and books that were priced to sell to a large public. My books had not become more academic. I have only written one kind of book, which is aimed at academics and the educated public.

One consequence of the decline in trade book interest was a decline as well in books that tried to take the measure of broad and unwieldy topics, of which health care is a prime example—in short, the kinds of books l wrote for Simon & Schuster between 1986 and 1998, numbering four in all, which were widely read and sold well. The decline in newspapers and magazines that review books has hardly helped. Books popularizing science still seem to sell well, particularly if they are exciting stories about the coming cure of cancer and Alzheimer's. But that approach is getting harder and harder for books in bioethics and health policy. Trade books on ethics, philosophical or theological, are almost nonexistent, neither sought by publishers nor blessed by university tenure committees. It is a noncategory in publishing, save by university presses, and for classroom use, not the general public. A 400-page dense study of ethics, assignable in college courses and selling for $50–$60, will not be found in most Barnes & Noble stores, much less in paperback in otherwise well-stocked airport book stores.

# 7

## The Future of Bioethics

Over the years I have been asked countless times about the future of bioethics. I have rarely had a good answer. That uncharacteristic loss of words was because I was thinking only of uncertain trends and projections; my crystal ball is small and cloudy. Yet there is another way to look at the future: trying to determine what it ought to be. That just takes some imagination and, if combined with some plausible predictions, might bear fruit. I will try to do just that. To do so, I will have to assess how well the field itself has done. Where are we now and where might we best go in the future?

A few broad strokes will set the stage. In the late 1960s, as bioethics was being born, there were only a few people teaching and writing on medical ethics. The term bioethics had not yet been coined. Until the Hastings Center came along in 1969, no institutions focused on it either. Only the Catholic medical schools and a scattering of secular schools offered a course on medical ethics. Now every medical school has one, and many have good-sized centers and programs. Bioethics is a popular undergraduate subject as well, and it would be hard to find a university that does not at least include some bioethics study, either as stand-alone courses or as part of other courses, usually biology, science and society, philosophy, and religion. A few schools offer a Ph.D. in bioethics, and many others offer an M.A. or a certificate of some kind (often appealing to physicians, nurses, and other health care professionals who wish to complement their main education and skills). Summer workshops are common. Every large university has an IRB, and often more than one, and hospital ethics committees are numerous. There is an international bioethics professional association and, in the United States, the American Society of Bioethics and Humanities often draws over 1,000 attendees at its annual meeting.

There have been five federal bioethics commissions or councils over the years, beginning in the mid-1970s and continuing into the Obama era. The media regularly publish articles on leading debates, and federal and state courts (and the Supreme Court) have made many decisions that resolve some of them. Internationally, every European country, some in the Middle East, Japan, China, and Singapore all display a wide range of bioethical activities. There are many American and international journals. What began more than forty years ago is now a well-established, thriving field.

## The Influence of Bioethics

How successful and influential has the field been? As for the success of the field—which did not begin with grand ambitions or a future picture anywhere approaching the extent to which it caught on and took root— one judgment seems sound. It significantly helped to establish the legitimacy of ethics as a field inside and outside of the academy, overcoming (for the most part) suspicion and even hostility about its value as a way of looking at ordinary life, much less scientific, medical, and professional practices. At a time when philosophy as a discipline is declining in universities, the teaching of bioethics has in many places kept alive ethical inquiry. Its acceptance in medical schools after the 1970s was itself a victory after an era of positivist triumphalism, banishing ethics to the outer darkness of emotivism and installing science as the emperor of the rationalist kingdom.

Beyond that victory, judgment becomes more difficult. There is good evidence that work in bioethics has had a place in the development of important government and professional codes and regulations. It has helped thousands of students better understand the challenges and dilemmas of biological and medical advances, in their own lives and that of society. It has helped bring ethical problems of importance to the attention of researchers and clinicians. It has had an important place in advancing the protection of important human rights, in human subject research, in the doctor-patient relationship, and the equitable distribution of health care resources. If many of the problems of bioethics are difficult and uncomfortable to talk about, it has brought most of them out from underground into the open air, worth considering, and fruitfully so.

But there are two questions worth pursuing. Apart from its ubiquity and academic popularity, what is its intellectual status, and how might we think about its future?

## The Intellectual Status of Bioethics

For many years, I have wondered about the intellectual status of bioethics. By that I mean the seriousness with which it is taken in university life and by the reading class outside of the university. That question has lurked in the back of my mind since the beginning, by which I mean the 1960s. It was a shock to discover when I arrived in New York in 1961 as a newcomer to the community of writers and journalists, that philosophy had little if any intellectual standing. History did, literature did, science did, cultural studies did, and surely politics did. Few philosophers broke into those circles, far fewer gained some ascendancy, and too often college philosophy courses were recalled as boring and technical. The notion that moral philosophy could be a source of knowledge and insight seemed nonexistent.

That experience helped me clarify my criteria for measuring the influence of bioethics. Our ideal at the Hastings Center was to attract an audience of clinicians and scientists, humanities and social science academics, and the educated public. We did not think of this as an idiosyncratic Hastings Center goal. We wanted well-grounded research that was interesting and accessible for the public. Though we were not aware of it at the time, it became evident that many free-standing research centers and "think tanks," many in Washington, had a similar goal (notably the Brookings Institution and the Urban Institute—but different from Heritage, Cato, and AEI, which have an aggressive and explicitly ideological agenda).

Toward that end, we sought to get our books published by prominent trade—not academic—publishers and our articles in such magazines as *Harper's*, the *Atlantic Monthly*, the *New York Times Magazine*, and the *New Republic* and as op-ed pieces in leading newspapers. We succeeded— but also got research articles published in the *New England Journal of Medicine* and the *Journal of the American Medical Association*. Meanwhile, the media flooded us with requests for comments and interviews. All in all, it was just what we wanted: a good balance of the academic and public. But it was a balance that neither the Hastings Center nor the field sustained, and maybe could not have sustained. The reasons are many, and will emerge as we move along. I want to begin with a basic question: what is our intellectual standing at present?

Among the high-level magazines in this country—for instance, the *New Yorker*, the *New York Review of Books*, the *Nation*, the *New Republic*, *Atlantic*, *Harper's*—articles on bioethics have been all but nonexistent in recent years, and few of us have ever been invited to write for them. Now and then topics pertinent to bioethics appear—for instance, synthetic biology in the *New Yorker*—but are usually not presented as ethical issues. It is no less rare for the mainline magazines and newspapers that run book reviews to review books on bioethics. It has been at least twelve years since the *New York Times Book Review* has reviewed a bioethics book (and that was a book of mine, *False Hopes*), and it was rare before that. Ironically, the field has attracted attention in some important conservative periodicals—the *Weekly Standard*, the *National Review*, and *Commentary*—but always to be attacked as a threat to morality, not a help.

The primary publishers of bioethics books—Oxford, Cambridge, MIT, and Georgetown, for instance—rarely if ever feature those books among those aimed at a larger reader public. I once asked a long-time bioethics editor at Oxford about that. He said those books are seen by the press as "niche" books, mainly of interest to those in the field and likely to be bought only for academic or classroom use. Three university presses have published my books, and none made it on to their general trade lists. My former editor at Simon & Schuster, who had published four of my books, told me in 1998 that my topics were simply not appealing to the large trade audience they sought and that she could publish me no more. My last book with her sold only 5,000 copies. My more recent books were effectively demoted to the academic presses.

So far as I know, only one person in bioethics—James Childress—has been elected a member of the American Philosophical Society, probably the country's most preeminent intellectual group (founded by Benjamin Franklin and, despite the name, not a philosophical society). The second most important such group is the American Academy of Arts and Science in Cambridge, and I know of only one person from bioethics who is a member—Alan Brandt. The number of bioethicists nominated for and elected to membership in the Institute of Medicine of the National Academy of Sciences, and to its governing council, has gradually declined over the years. The 1970s and 1980s were the peak years.

We have all been aware for many years that only a few foundations include bioethics among their stated areas of interest, and not one of the major health care foundations does. To be sure, we have received a good deal of money over the years from the private foundations, but that has usually been because we could show our pertinence to one of their established philanthropy areas, which was often a stretch at that. Although I heard scattered stories over the years about wealthy individual benefactors helping a few bioethics centers (notably Johns Hopkins and ours, only recently), it seems relatively rare.

For those raising money for either ours or other bioethics organizations, my experience has been that, given the ambiguous, faintly skeptical understanding of ethics as a field of inquiry by many, it is wise to use our issues as the primary drawing card and to place the field of ethics itself in a secondary role. It is easier, in short, to show the importance of the problems we take on than that our field, ethics, has the intellectual tools and skills to handle them. I believe that is a false judgment, but for those primarily drawn to bottom-line, decisive outcomes of research and inquiry—a common characteristic of many wealthy people—it needs to be taken into account. They did not make their money by reflecting on the nature and future of human life under the influence of scientific ambition, a basic and enduring matter for bioethics.

I offer the above information less as a "why don't they love us more" lament than out of a kind of curiosity. We all get speaking invitations and invitations to take part in important meetings and conferences, national and international. As an institution we have a high standing, as do others, in bioethics. We are a major source of information for the media—and our issues have a high profile. Yet we, and just about everyone in the field, have not made it to the American intellectual first team—or to the second string. Peter Singer is a notable exception. At best, only a handful of bioethicists have had any status at all in the national health care debate, full of ethical struggles (even if not so labeled). As it might be put in the movie business, we have all had a few small speaking parts and cameo roles, but not much more. The gap between the wide range of activities noted above and the intellectual status of the field is wide. Let me try to offer some reasons.

I noted in an early chapter how the routinization of charisma affected me in the 1980s, recalling that old social science concept about how organizations and institutions usually move from their exciting startup days to a steadier but more routine and less exciting life as they age. Despite a fair degree of skepticism or hostility to bioethics in some quarters in the 1970s, there was also a matching enthusiasm in others. The issues were new, the field was fresh, and public interest in it all was new as well. The field and the Center attracted attention, not just its issues (unlike the present time when the two seem reversed), and expectations were high. We made no efforts whatever to reach out to the media, but they came to us in droves.

## The Glamour Fades, the Field Grows

As time went on, the excitement died down. However, as the field faded a bit at the public level, it grew at the academic level. It turned out that the field did not have big answers to big questions, but some useful things to say about some things; soon people and fields other than bioethics began having their say on the issues also. Those in the field of bioethics (which still has fuzzy boundaries) gradually ceased being the sole commentator on bioethics. Doctors with no background in ethics are as likely to be interviewed on ethics as those of us who think about it as a profession—and do just as well.

The glamour was mainly gone by the end of the 1980s, just as in universities the glitter of the new subspecialties of black studies, women's studies, American and urban studies soon gave way to academic routinization. When was the last time you saw any media attention paid to those programs, the darlings of the media in the 1970s and 1980s? Bioethics had by then moved well down the road to becoming an academic subdiscipline, shifting in a radical way the earlier balance between the academic and the popular.

Although excessive hostility (or worse, tepidity) was often matched by enthusiasm in the early years, there remains a wide range of opinion on the value of ethics as a professional field. One does not have to scratch far below the surface in most medical schools to find either indifference, or even some hostility, to ethics (often directed at IRBs and their bureaucratization of ethics) taken to be soft and mushy against the transcendent value of hard scientific knowledge.

Even at a theoretical level, as a recent issue of the old and internationally distinguished British journal *Philosophy* made evident, philosophy itself is rent with arguments about just what it is in the first place, and what difference—if any—it makes in the second place. Moral philosophy comes off no better than epistemology, logic, and the philosophy of mind. All are being away nipped at by science, stealing away many traditional philosophical subjects and by a public—even an educated one—that is not impressed with the field. Bioethics may be one of its bright spots, even as an early dominance by philosophers seems to be fading.

The field of bioethics has, in short, a peculiar combination of issues that are of the greatest importance and public interest but that are also embedded in a field that many, inside and outside of the academy, are less than impressed by. How can one beat aging, death, health and illness, designer babies and genetic engineering, human enhancement, and the relief of pain and suffering for basic human interest? But how can the field that takes on those matters rise above its hybrid nature, the mixed judgment in the academy on its value, the varying verdict of the public on it, and its seemingly endless, unresolved arguments (on enhancement, brain death, and the limits to autonomy, for instance)?

To add to those challenges, moral philosophy—even as a well-established academic and intellectual field—has its share of troubles as well. *Philosophy* regularly publishes articles attempting to deal with the plethora of competing ethical theories at the most basic level and with what, exactly, ethics is all about. Has there been progress in its 2,500 or so years? You can get more than one answer, and more likely twenty, to that question from philosophers.

## The Progress of Bioethics

Has bioethics made progress in its forty or fifty years of existence? Yes and no. Yes, in the sense that some arguments, issues, and policies have been refined over the years. I said "refined," not solved. The definition of death, one of our very first issues, would be a case in point. The "whole brain" concept of death seems on its way out, but there is more than one contender to take its place. Care at the end of life, and the termination of treatment, which initially did not look all that hard, has made some progress but the discussion sounds at least 80 percent the same now as forty years ago. The discussions at 2010 meetings of our synthetic biology group did not sound too different from those that accompanied the controversial recombinant DNA research of the 1970s. How are risks and benefits best balanced?

It may well be the case that, like the field of ethics itself, ever changing since the time of Plato and Aristotle (but still finding them insightful), the issues of bioethics will never be fully resolved and put to one side but always transmuting because of new scientific knowledge and further thought on central ethical questions. In fact, it is hard to think of any bioethical problem that will get definitively solved and be put aside. At the least, new generations will come along with different histories from ours, different scientific and cultural perspectives, and different social contexts. They may not have to start afresh but they may well find that what we have bequeathed to them is not sufficient for their needs.

I have never believed in the idea that in our pluralistic societies, there can be no fixed and forever valid moral principles. I believe we have many values in common. The difficult challenge is trying to make sense of and live up to them, in changing historical times and with ever-changing scientific information in culturally shifting societies. That can be done, but it will always be a struggle.

## A Lack of Rigor?

The main and most persistent criticism, however, is that too much scholarship and writing in bioethics is not careful and "rigorous" enough. Usually, if not always, this criticism comes from people in the standard disciplines. For philosophers, their charge is that there is insufficient analytical precision and well-wrought arguments in bioethics. For social scientists, their judgment is either that the common mode of bioethical analysis is weak on empirical grounding or insufficiently attentive to the cultural and social context of bioethical problems. For physicians, the accusation is that bioethicists are too often naïve or ignorant about clinical realities.

Off and on over the years, there has been criticism of bioethicists, at least some of them, that they are too quick and glib with sound bites for the media. From conservatives have come complaints that bioethics is, at base, liberal, excessively secular, and not open to conservative perspectives. Liberals have taken shots at conservatives in return. Finally, there have been comments over the years by nonacademic members of the Center's board of directors that too much writing by bioethicists is technical and impenetrable for lay people.

There is something to all of those criticisms. Interdisciplinary work has no well-established criteria for rigor, although I believe most of us in the field can distinguish good work from bad. I would also note that those who write in the field from a strictly rigorous disciplinary perspective usually have little influence outside of their discipline. And the audience for bioethics is made up of many disciplines. Those who are most influential manage, in their writing, to transcend the style of those in their own discipline. Those too wedded to their discipline and its characteristic style of analysis and discourse are likely to lose a lay audience, even a well-educated one.

As for the charges about sound bites and the media, there is little way to control that. All of us have the experience of giving long interviews to reporters writing a story and having them reduced to one sentence, usually the most trivial one we utter. If one of the goals of the field is to reach out to the public, not just students and other academics, then we must talk ordinary nondisciplinary language and take our chances with the media. And, yes, the field is moderately liberal in its persuasions, but also liberal in the sense of a willingness to listen to the other side, even if not often enough. A tendency to clannishness among conservatives has led them to be happier talking with each other than mixing it up with liberals. Both sides can take some blame for the culture wars. The larger polarities of America culture have made their way into bioethics.

## What Are We Trying to Do?

I conclude with a basic question, with the field since the start and never fully answered: just what should those of in the field be trying to do, and what kind of person ought we be in order to best do it? I put to one side the kind of Never Never Land answer that I received as a graduate student in the late 1950s at Harvard: the aim of good ethics is, intellectually, what results from independence, rationality, impersonality, and emotional detachment—an ideal observer. The kind of person one should be to achieve those aims, moreover, has nothing to do with one's moral character. It is a matter of philosophical rigor, intelligence, knowledge of the field and its debates, clever thought experiments, and quickness with good counterarguments. The skills necessary to be a good chess player offer an analogy, particularly love of it as a game of wits.

I should in fairness qualify that judgment by noting that metaethics was in the saddle in those days, that of a focus not on ethical judgments and principles but on ethical theory and conceptual analysis. Normative ethics, at least for the moment, had been pushed aside, not to reappear until the late 1960s and 1970s. Even so, many of the traits and proclivities of that era still linger on, too often guaranteeing that forms of language and argumentation of interest only to other philosophers (or other bioethicists for that matter) that block public accessibility and influence. But then those virtues are not likely to help young academics to gain tenure and grants (and interdisciplinary skills are not too helpful, either). A modern day variant on John Stuart Mills's classic essay "On Liberty"—clear, concise, and accessible to anyone who can read—stands in naked contrast to Immanuel Kant's *Critique of Pure Reason*, which has none of those traits but is nonetheless a classic also. I doubt, however, that Mills's essay—a perfect op-ed piece in writing style—is even now held up as a model for disciplinary writers, whatever the field, but it surely should be for bioethicists.

### Aiming for Influence

Not only should the literature of bioethics be interdisciplinary, requiring of necessity accessibility to those in disciplines other than that of the author, but it should aim no less to have public, clinical, and policy influence. Sometimes we will want to have a conversation among ourselves, or write something for our colleagues. But it should not be the rule, much less the test of a successful career. It should not be held against a philosopher for publishing in a medical journal an article with somewhat less nuance than he or she might display in a philosophical journal; the rule that no sentence should have to be read twice is pertinent here. Nor should publishing op-ed articles fail to count toward tenure.

As someone who has failed more often than not in getting a piece accepted in a major newspaper, it is a far more competitive arena than that of peer-reviewed journals. It requires the most demanding of all norms: one must have something original and significant to say, and then say it with some flair and complete lucidity. I note in passing, not altogether sure what to make of it, that conservative bioethicists have a pronounced tendency to use the unreferenced essay, not too long, as its main means of communication. Long, scholarly books, heavy with footnotes, are rare, as are its articles in that academic mode. The Bush administration's President's Council did not start with them but came to include a list of pertinent bioethics articles as part of their reports. But there is little evidence of their influence the contents of those reports. I do not mean that aside to be necessarily disparaging. They were marching to a different drummer; the bioethics literature did not speak to their hearts, and the readable, unfootnoted essay style, for reports or articles, often has a better chance of gaining an audience. I like some of my short essays as much as my scholarly books, and I know that many of them have had a wider readership.

## Enduring Issues

When the Hastings Center decided in its early days to sharpen its focus, we chose issues we believed would be enduring in the coming years: death and dying, behavior control, population and reproductive biology, and genetics. Our foresight proved to be accurate. We might well have added human subject research to that list. And here is where I can make a prediction: not one of them is likely to go away. They will be affected by new scientific knowledge, social and medical needs, fresh cadres of researchers and clinicians, and the simple fact that all of them touch at some deep level on ancient and enduring ethical, legal, and political problems, never once and for all solved.

Our first major research project was on brain death, and we accepted the general consensus at the time that death occurs with "the irreversible cessation of all functions of the entire brain, including the brainstem," or the "irreversible cessation of circulatory and respiratory functions."

At first we discussed when biological death occurs: all at once or only gradually? We came to find that no ready agreement existed on that matter. We then asked a different question—what condition would be sufficient to legally declare a patient dead—and whole brain death was the answer. In a few short years, every state accepted that definition, and it still stands. But there have always been critics, many in bioethics. I have come to accept the judgment of one who is herself a bioethicist, Tia Powell, that bioethicists' criticism "have proved irrelevant to health policy . . . [and] that there is more pressing work to do than to seek perfection in the definition of death." But I doubt that will happen. I should add that our later work focused on death itself as pertinent to end-of-life care (which I will return to shortly), and that latter issue, seemingly solved in theory by the end of the 1970s, has continued to this day.

The population limitation focus of the 1960s gradually declined as changes in international UN policy and falling global birthrates came to pass (save for sub-Saharan Africa). It was replaced, however, in the 1990s by population birthrates well below the replacement rate (2.1 children per women) in all the developed countries (save for the United States) but especially in Italy, Greece, Spain, Poland, Korea, Japan, and China). Those developments have received little attention in the United States, though there has remained to this day a hardy group of demographers and environmentalists who welcome the decline on environmental grounds. Unlike population problems, assisted reproduction has been another matter in the United States, with the advent of sperm and egg donation, surrogate motherhood, and particularly the use of those techniques by single women and gay couples.

Our interest in behavior control by surgical, drug, and behavioral modification had declined by the 1980s as psychosurgery, much criticized, more or less vanished and other earlier-touted techniques came to offer little promise. By the mid-2000s, however, it came back with new forms of psychosurgery (e.g., deep brain stimulation for epileptics) and the outbreak of a major debate on the under- and overuse of pharmaceuticals in the treatment of children. In 2011 I wandered into the obesity debate, asking whether social stigma is ethically acceptable way of changing the behavior of the obese (my answer: a decisive maybe). But obesity falls into a class of problems that will probably expand in the future: public health problems that require change in ways of life and behavior.

As for genetics, its advances have produced a cornucopia of ethical challenges, from the recombinant DNA fights of the 1970s, through the genome mapping effort of the 1980s and 1990s, to the present struggle over synthetic biology. Along the way have come prenatal diagnosis, newborn genetic screening, stem cell research, presymptomatic adult screening for adult-onset disease, and sex selection. Those developments will continue indefinitely to pose ethical challenges. Human subject research, our final early area, is still being refined, and endless tinkering with IRB regulations go on as ever (and the regulations always grow in size). The concept of informed consent, the core moral requirement for ethical research, may even surpass the definition of death for sustained tinkering.

If those have been enduring issues for bioethics, the meat and potatoes of the field, they have been matched by the pervasiveness of some long-standing root problems at a different level. They represent what I think of as enduring tensions: individual good and common good, ethics and the law, professional self-regulation and government regulation, risks and benefits, universal ethical principles and cultural particularities, the scope and limits of autonomy, the "is" and the "ought," essentialist and nonessentialist notions of human nature and human dignity, and the right and the good.

A whole category of what might be called the bioethics service industry will no doubt endure. The most common are IRBs and hospital ethics committees. They serve large numbers of people and provide a necessary base for some important ethical analysis well outside of the public eye.

In this section and the next, I will look at two cultures: medicine and biology and that of bioethics. It is the interaction of these ever-changing cultures that helps to define the field, setting its agenda and shaping its response to constant medical and technological advances. These changes have dovetailed with a rise in affluence since World War II (itself a cause of higher health care demand and costs), a heightened quest for personal freedom (blending a libertarian-inclined left and a market-oriented right: choice as the common currency), and a change of mores in public and private life (intensified by the media and the social network).

## The Culture of Medicine

Although not an exclusive one by any means, a useful task for bioethics in the future will be a careful analysis of the downstream effects of the medical and biological advances. What have those advances brought, and which have been good, bad, or mixed in their impact? Many of the early years of the field focused on the likely ethical problems of newly emergent scientific advances and technology, and that will surely remain true in the future. But to better understand where we have come from, and how things have turned out, will help to determine what ought to be changed or reversed, and now better to assess the advances of the future.

I have found it useful over the years to think about three features of the culture of medicine: changes in the way that culture has come to think about medicine itself, in its understanding of health and disease, and how it has come to change the way we think about living a life.

## Changes in the Meaning and Scope of Health and Disease

In the early years of the field, a number of articles and anthologies examined the concepts of health, disease, sickness, and disease. An article of mine criticizing the World Health Organization (WHO) definition of health has been periodically been reprinted for close to forty years, and Arthur Caplan was a prominent and insightful contributor to that literature. I am not certain what difference, if any, those mainly theoretical and conceptual analyses made at the clinical or policy level, and they gradually faded away. They were superseded by a spotlight turned on the growing phenomenon of medicalization, an issue that overlapped with complaints about the power of the pharmaceutical industry in shaping public and physician attitudes about health and illness.

Medicalization can be defined, in my reading, as the phenomenon of turning into treatable medical conditions once-ordinary and seemingly unavoidable pains, illnesses, and threats to life and health. Put in a slightly different way, whatever feature of our lives, physical or mental, that disturbs us can be turned into a medical problem if some way can be found to treat medically treat it, sometimes because what was a real, acknowledged problem can now be treated, and sometimes because we just don't like it (pattern baldness).

My favorite anecdote of the former kind comes from the Czech Republic in the early 1990s. I asked a geriatrician there how Alzheimer's disease was treated in her country. Her answer was that it is neither diagnosed nor treated, it is just accepted as part of getting old (we all get forgetful as we age). I was astonished by that answer, coming from a country where statistically Alzheimer's was rapidly becoming a dread disease to compete with cancer for attention.

That story had what I call an O'Henry ending. A few years later I asked my informant if there had been any new developments with Alzheimer's. "Yes," she said, "we now have an active committee looking at the issue and working to get it diagnosed and treated by physicians." How had that happened, I asked? The Pfizer Company had put up the money for the committee, in great part to sell its drug Aricept (expensive and of only marginal value). That same informant, by the way, came to enjoy a great boost to her abysmally low income as a physician by organizing clinical trials for drug companies (with great ethical care).

Medicalization continues to move along at a fast pace, fueled by drug and device companies looking for new markets and making aggressive use of direct-to-consumer advertising. The media is a helpful enabler, very ready to announce in a celebratory way new breakthroughs and promising research. If the United States has not quite become a nation of hypochondriacs, it may be well on its way. Joining the enthusiasts are a fair number of bioethicists who contend that aging itself, and not just the pathologies that go with it, is medically treatable and those who say there is no great inherent difference between ordinary medical therapies and radical enhancement efforts, it is a movement of medicine along a seamless continuum.

## Changes in the Way We Live Our Lives

This category is the one where the downstream effects of medical progress require the most analysis. I will simply list them and raise some questions worth future pursuit and being too little examined now. In many instances, they require a questioning of the status quo, where routinization and habituation have dulled critical faculties.

I have long believed the following to be a true axiom: every medical advance in the name of expanded individual choice and freedom will most likely settle into a socially shaped routine expectation, sometimes coercively so. Predictive and personalized medicine, for instance, have opened up the possibility of considerable foreknowledge of our future health risks. We now have a choice between taking advantage of that knowledge or ignoring it. But just as prenatal diagnosis has become as routine as the taking of blood pressure, we would be wise to expect that the choice to use predictive medicine will give way to an expectation that of course we should take advantage of it. Our individual and public health will seem to require it.

## Longer Life Spans

Save for sub-Saharan Africa, international birthrates steadily declined during the twentieth century, with many countries experiencing rates well below the replacement level. Even so, the seven billion mark was passed not long ago. If excessively high birthrates (seven or more children) were a problem for poor countries, very low birthrates pose a different kind of challenge for developed countries, creating a severe pension and social security burden as well as high health care costs. Meanwhile some environmentalists and demographers believe that although there are some high social costs, low birthrates are a necessity in developed countries because of the environmental impact of the affluent lifestyle that has accompanied their economic growth. What is a reasonable goal for birthrates in developed countries? How should would-be parents think about the social implications of their childbearing desires? What kind of social obligations do those who chose to have none, or no more than one or two children, have to use their affluence responsibly to meet environmental needs? How far and in what way should governments go to raise, if such they are judged to be, excessively low birthrates?

A drop in infant mortality rates beginning in the nineteenth century was the first determinant of increased life expectancy. The second was an increase over the past forty years of some eight or nine years in life expectancy beyond the age of 65, a change that together with lower birth rates in developed countries has meant a hazardous change in the dependency ratios, with fewer young workers to support a growing number of retirees. It has no less meant that an overwhelming number of elderly will end their lives with expensive chronic illnesses, often marked by insufficient retirement income.

While bioethicists have wrestled with the cost problem and questions of equity in resource allocation, three large questions have been relatively neglected. First, how can personal meaning and a revised social role for the elderly be conceptualized, developed, and implemented? Second, in light of the cost issue, how can resources for the critically ill—but not necessarily imminently dying—elderly be made more affordable and sustainable? Third, how can the burden of family care for the elderly, especially the demented, be made more equitable and tolerable, both within the family and or with the help of outside services?

## Behavior Control in a New Key

As noted earlier, early emphasis was on the use of technology to change and manipulate behavior, and some of that kind of research still goes on. Of somewhat more recent vintage are a number of efforts to improve or decisively change the behavior of those who health and living habits are a cause of bad health. My late-1960s foray into family planning policy aiming to lower birthrates showed how important, and often ethically problematic, such efforts can be. More recently campaigns to reduce teen age pregnancies, HIV/AIDS, smoking, and obesity moved into public view. As I discovered while writing a 2011 article on the use of stigma as a public health tactic to reduce obesity, it is a volatile and sensitive topic for obesity experts and the obese themselves. Is it ethical to deliberately stigmatize the elderly, as was done with smokers as part of the antismoking campaign? How far can law and regulation go to control the sale of known contributors to obesity, such as high sugar and fructose products? How much power should employers have to use economic incentives and disincentives in affecting obesity-related behavior among their employees?

In my book *Taming the Beloved Beast*, I developed an argument that the classic individual-oriented model of clinical medicine needed to be balanced by a competitive public health mode and to often override that former model. I criticized the Medicare standard of providing benefits solely on the basis of a standard of "reasonable and necessary." That standard, I noted, has always been vague and difficult to apply—the words "reasonable" and "necessary" shot through with ambiguity and problems of interpretation. Most important, they were deliberately intended by Congress to forestall and deny any consideration of cost, the fruits of active lobbying by medical and industry forces.

Is a $100,000 cancer treatment that provides only a few extra weeks of life reasonable and necessary? I argue that such a question should be answered by the use of a population, not individual, standard: does it make a contribution to population health and cost control? That is an unavoidable question for future research. As part of my thesis, I contended that we should think about the needs of different age groups, not of individuals in those groups, as a basis for research allocation, concluding that the elderly have a weaker claim on health care resource than children or working age adults.

## Pregnancy and Childbearing

Although the likely success of Robert Edwards and Patrick Steptoe in developing successful in vitro fertilization (IVF) was uncertain at the time and already controversial before they succeeded in 1974 with Louise Brown, I don't believe anyone foresaw just how massive its effects would be. In its own right and in conjunction with sperm and egg donation and surrogate motherhood, it has relieved millions of cases of the infertility of married couples and has also made possible childbearing for single women and gay partners. It has no less made possible late procreation for women over the age of 35—but at the price of twins, triplets, and beyond for many; some risk to the mother's health; increased infant mortality; and some dashed hopes by women who delayed pregnancy, expecting that IVF would work for them—but the odds of success decline with age.

The issues that have most come to my mind are three. Would it better if women returned to childbearing in their 20s and early 30s, reducing the need for IVF, and what kinds of career and work patterns and social and policy policies could make that attractive and feasible? What will be the long-term success of the multiple procreational arrangements and their impact on children, well worth following—and no less with deliberately single parents? What is the importance of a biological relationship?

I will say something only about that last question. As noted earlier, I am an opponent of sperm and egg donation, especially when it is said that the donor has no parental responsibility for the outcome. It seems to me a gross misuse of procreational freedom. But a common response has been that a biological relationship is not necessary for a good parent-child relationship; love and care are the main need—donors are thus irrelevant. But donors are wanted, are they not, because the recipient prizes a biological relationship, and that is considered an acceptable desire, isn't it? And of late, both with adoption and sperm/egg donation, there has been a small but growing movement to ban sperm/egg donation or, if it is allowed to continue, to give to children the right to know who the donor was and to seek them out if desired.

So, does biology count? It will surely count in the development of diagnostic screening programs, hunting for genetic or other markers of disease predispositions, which will be among the most troubling medical technologies in the years to come. Knowing the genetic background of donors is already important, but it will become more so with ordinary marital procreation between a fertile man and woman as well. And the common desire of adopted children and those procreated with sperm and egg donations—although strictly speaking, it proves nothing about the biological relationship—is surely suggestive and not easy to ignore.

Over the past few decades, enormous changes have taken place in the bearing and rearing of children. Those changes began with more effective contraception, notably the birth control pill, and then came medically safer legal abortion in 1973. An efficacious choice of whether to have a baby, and how many and with what spacing, became a reality. The term "designer babies" became popular as procreational choice was extended, at least hypothetically, to choosing children's genetic traits. Prenatal diagnosis moved along rapidly, eventually including sex selection, followed most recently by a growing range of postnatal screening possibilities, the outer limit of which is nowhere in sight.

Parents will know more and more about their children's possibilities and probabilities for early- and late-onset diseases. Running in parallel with those developments have been advances in drugs and their application to children with mild and severe mental health problems, now a conflicted area of research and clinical application. I was astonished when my granddaughter returned from camp one summer to report that every child she came to know there was taking pills for something or other. She was the exception. And despite this not being a medical problem as such, the impact of the social media on children has been enormous, with considerable uncertainty about its long-term influence on their intellectual and emotional life. It is already thought to be a factor (along with TV and electronic games) in the rise of childhood obesity.

In light of the new possibilities, some basic questions need increased attention. How should we think about childhood, now expanded to encompass adolescence and early adulthood? What kinds of choices that parents can and sometimes must make about their child's future will be good or harmful? Parents have always had the familial power of shaping their children's lives to a considerable degree, as well as wittingly or unwittingly doing harm to them. Now they have medical and genetic power as well. What is a good balance between parental hopes and desires and power and the need for children to grow up as their own unique persons, not manipulated in their parent's image? How is the knowledge that predictive medicine will bring to be deployed and wisely used? And should it be welcomed in the first place?

## The Culture of Bioethics

As a now-established academic subspecialty, how might we best under-stand the culture of bioethics? Even a glance at the disciplinary range of those who contribute to the *Hastings Center Report* shows its interdis-ciplinarity, and the same could be said for other journals. Contributors come from a wide range of disciplines: media studies, philosophy, nursing, medicine, political science, religious studies, health policy, hos-pital chaplaincy, law, psychology, sociology, and anthropology. No one traditional discipline has a leading role. The earlier domination of field first by theology then later by philosophy appears to have faded—in fact, physicians seem to be somewhat in the ascendancy now. The one field strikingly absent is economics (paralleled by the dominance of economists and empirically oriented policy analysts in the major health care foundations, notably and perennially disinterested in bioethics). And although I call bioethics an academic subspecialty, I would qualify that characterization by noting that many writers, researchers, and clinicians are not academics or only partly so (e.g., clinical professors of medicine who may teach an ethics course or serve on an IRB or hospital ethics committee).

But it is an academic subspecialty by some common standards: peer-reviewed journals and the listings of grants in CVs—and there are some difficulties with professional assessments where the university or medical standards are usually disciplinary (for instance, a philosopher with an appointment in a department of surgery). Moreover, there are a number of subspecialties in bioethics, even though many in the field shift around from time to time or mix them together. Each requires different disciplinary skills, often well beyond someone's original and traditional discipline. **Clinical ethics** requires familiarity with the methods and ethos of medical decision making, medical language and concepts, end-of-life care, and the doctor-patient relationship. **Research ethics** and IRB service need an understanding of research methods and protocols, legal rules and regulations on human subject research, and ethical insight into the recruitment and retention of research subjects. **Health policy ethics** requires familiarity with health economics, policy science, health care regulations, and quantitative policy analysis. **Cultural bioethics** requires an understanding of the role of culture, professional mores, and political and social ideologies, in shaping background values and ethical predilections. **Public health ethics** concentrates on disease and epidemic surveillance, health improvement and disease prevention, and socioeconomic determinants of health.

Two more recent subspecialties have emerged of late. One of them might be called **political bioethics**, by which I do not mean a focus on such traditional health care topics as resource allocation, priority setting, and deliberative democracy but instead a focus on the clash of ideological values, which always have ethical ingredients, and on the "dirty hands" work of political compromise and the tailoring of ethical principles to political realities. The other is that of the **biological and evolutionary foundations of morality**, which has only a few bioethical followers (and some believe it has little to contribute to normative ethics). Obviously knowledge of genetics and biological and evolutionary theory is needed here. I have left out a few that are important also: global health ethics and organizational ethics, for instance, and some advocate for a rights-based bioethics.

## The Methods of Bioethics

Some years ago, I tried to formulate some criteria for interdisciplinary bioethics. It is the need to have a foundation in a traditional discipline, to have an eye out for the ramifications of an ethical problem in other disciplines, and, if a particular subfield is being pursued, to become a competent amateur in another discipline. My core discipline is philosophy, but in writing my book *Medicine and the Market*, I had to become a competent amateur in the history of market theories in medicine and western industrial societies, health care economics, and the politics and ideologies of market versus government strategies in managing health care systems. I could by no means always understand the economic methodologies in health care, much less evaluate them in particular contexts (particularly when the acknowledged experts disagreed). But I could at least grasp and follow the logic of their arguments and often use my philosophical skills of analysis to bring a different angle of vision, and often criticism to their debates. It does take a certain intellectually adventurous bent to do that sort of thing (and an ever-present anxiety about possible humiliations for saying dumb or, even worse, trivial things—the only good antidote for which is to ask an expert to read a draft to make sure there are no obvious gaffes or banalities).

Just as I learned how complicated, messy, and uncertain clinical medicine could be in trying to blend the art and science of care, I also found most of the serious ethical problems, at the policy or clinical levels, not reducible to or easily amenable to the deployment of formal ethical theory. Trying to find a way, for instance, to deal with reciprocal generational duties between the young and the old while at the same time trying to determine how to fairly ration elderly Medicare benefits—all the while trying to take account of the revealed preferences of the elderly and their children whose taxes in a pay-as-you-go program pay for that care—tends to make a hash of conceptual tidiness. The best I can often come up with is Aristotelian prudence and soldiering on in the face of confusion, my own and everyone else's, keeping the large theories in the back of one's mind but never letting them call the shots in trying to grasp complex and multilayered ethical problems and dilemmas.

That much said, two troubling methodological issues need to be considered: the role of empirical evidence in bioethical analysis, and some untoward effects of policy analysis on the field. The former has been well noticed, but not quite fully, and the latter hardly at all. Except for a time in the late 1970s into the 1980s, when moral philosophy came to be the dominant discipline and rules, principles, and ethical theories the tools of choice, empirical bioethics has long had an expanding place, even if that phrase was not used. Early complaints by social scientists about the absence of their skills and knowledge in the fledgling field made a difference. As moral philosophy has faded from its dominance—hardly out of the picture but now often ignored or minimized by those trained in other fields—empirical evidence and modes of analysis have become common, notably in studies of human subject research, end-of-life care, and childbearing. That is an important development and one that is surely valuable in defining issues, situating them in their social context, and testing (where feasible) their reflection of human and medical experience. Those features offer a useful counterbalance to philosophy's tendency to impersonally large abstractions and fine distinctions. Johns Rawls's idea of a reflective equilibrium aims to catch that tension and dialectic.

## Empirical Bioethics and the Humanities

I have two worries here. One is the possibility of giving empirical perspectives a higher role than that of the humanities and, not unrelated, capitulating to scientists and policymakers for whom empirical perspectives and evidence are the sine qua non of good research. Proposals to the NIH to work on bioethical issues are often reviewed not by other bioethicists but by scientists in the disciplines most pertinent to the ethical problems. There is often both explicit and implicit pressure to sound as scientific as possible and to find and accentuate empirical angles and research as part of grant proposals. A leading bioethicist, Ezekiel Emanuel, once told the audience at an annual meeting of the American Society for Bioethics and Humanities that giving empirical issues a dominant role would be critical to the success of bioethical proposals.

Just that kind of advice threatens to minimize the important role of the humanities in bioethics. Although bioethics is, I would argue, essentially an interdisciplinary field, its roots lie in the humanities. Its central focus on ethics makes that clear, whether from a philosophical or theological perspective. But more than that, as I trust my earlier discussions of ethics reveal, I take seriously the often-mocked idea of wisdom, the very nature of which—as William James exemplified and as Socrates and Aristotle embodied—means taking account of the full range of human knowledge and experience: history, the physical and social sciences, religion, philosophy, literature, and cultural studies, among others. Thought experiments offer a way of avoiding that kind of complexity, making it possible to cut through all that while sitting at one's desk. Only philosophers, sitting in hot houses, could come up with such a clean way of dealing with life as it is, which was not designed for thought experiments.

To do good work in bioethics requires that one be widely read and something of a polymath (which I am surely not, but hopefully may be when I get older). My wife and I subscribe to twenty or so journals in at least ten disciplines. Although medical, health policy, and my wife's psychology and theology journals (despite my being an unbeliever) are imperative reading, I have also gained some useful ideas for bioethics from magazines and journals having nothing to do with those topics. The journal *Foreign Affairs* is notable for its absence of articles on medicine and biology, but full of insights on the solving of nasty policy problems. The journal *Technology and Society* rarely publishes anything on medical technology, but its articles on technology in other contexts contain many suggestive and transferable ideas. Much of my thinking on birthrates and aging has come from a thirty-year subscription to the journal *Population and Development Review*. The magazine *Science* is invaluable for its research articles (many of which are incomprehensible to nonspecialists), but no less for its reporting on the politics, financing, and mission of science. The *New Yorker*, the *New Republic*, the *New York Review of Books*, and the *Atlantic* are useful for their broad range of topics, but also as models of good, clear writing. I was once told that the best way to become a good writer is not necessarily to read books on that topic but to constantly read good writing, so that it sinks into one's consciousness and shapes the way one looks at language and its rhythms and possibilities.

## Ethics and Policy: Some Hidden Pitfalls

My other worry about the future of bioethics is the heavy emphasis on ethics and policy, one of its strengths but presenting some pitfalls. At the outset of the field, as described in chapter 3, there were two streams, one focused on the large questions of the potential impact of medical and biological advances on our conceptions of human nature and the living of a human life and the other stream centered on specific clinical and policy problems (especially human subject research). The earlier phase got drowned out by the latter and was not revived until George W. Bush's President's Council on Bioethics—which was then made fun of for doing so by many in bioethics, whose liberal ideology was as conspicuously visible from the left as was the Council's conservatism from the right. The heavy-handed announcement of the Obama Commission that its focus would be on ethics and policy came across as a deliberate rebuke to Bush's President's Council. It sought in effect to return to the status quo ante, considered the real stuff.

Surely there is nothing wrong with exploring the policy problems that bioethical issues generate. They matter, are important, and affect our lives. But an emphasis that treats policy issues as if they are the heart of our work carries some liabilities for ethics, the most obvious of which is the premium placed on finding politically acceptable compromises on contentious issues. Policy cannot be made without finding ways to bridge differences. Nor can policy be made by modes of analysis that drive the issues deeper and deeper into the realm of the aims, goals, and meaning of human life. Those who put together the UN Declaration of Human Rights in the aftermath of WWII were said to be able to agree on specific rights as long as they did not seek agreement on the disputed foundation for such rights. And the tradition of the U.S. Supreme Court is, so far as possible, to avoid going to the mat on deeply fundamental constitutional issues; better to avoid such problems by accepting, whenever possible, the decisions of lower courts.

The net result of policy work is not only a bias toward empirical work, readily pursued and popular in policy studies, but also putting to one side and out of sight fundamental questions of good and evil, right and wrong, virtues and vices—the very stuff at the historical foundation of ethics. Those are uncomfortable words for public policy (save in the most extreme circumstances), divisive and inflammatory, unsuitable (and often rightly so) for the policy work of consensus building and the accommodation of conflicting values and principles. The problem is how to keep alive and encourage ongoing consideration of those deeper matters, making certain they have at least a consideration in policy work—and enough vitality beyond it to keep them alive and influential. The President's Council put them on the front line, a valuable contribution, only to be to criticized for doing so. And their reports were equal in quality to any earlier presidential commission, just different.

### Assessing New Technologies

There is also another reason to be careful of at least some kinds of policy work, particularly the assessment of new technologies. Those technologies rarely appear on a level playing field—but are usually presented as if they are. New technologies are ordinarily developed and disseminated by large and powerful corporations or, just prior to that, a strong coalition of interested parties who want research on them to go forward. The $3 billion California stem cell research ballot initiative had behind it prominent scientists, media celebrities, legislators, and wealthy business interests—and a public reflexively ready to embrace medical research with much-touted health benefits in the offing. No citizen's group could have resisted that kind of clout, and none did despite ethical objections. That was the case earlier with recombinant DNA research, and now with synthetic biology. President Obama's Presidential Commission took on synthetic biology as its first project and issued a report at the end of 2010. Its work was carefully organized, open to all perspectives, and altogether a model of a presidential commission report. Its recommendation was also altogether predictable—move ahead but with caution and oversight—given its scientific support, the thrill of discovery, and the long list of potential benefits advanced by the researchers, every bit as expansive as those promised by the advent of stem cell research. The bottom line: no serious obstacles were put in the way of the research.

I am not here complaining that the commission did not take the critics seriously or was not thorough in its research. Those are not the issues that concern me. What does concern me is instead that the effort to craft a careful balance between excessive celebration and oppressive caution, history suggests, usually favors support of the research. That is the predictable outcome. It is always easier to say yes than no to medical progress in the United States, and the commission said yes.

We would do well to recall a constant refrain over the years that scientific and technological progress often outrun ethical solutions to the problems they raise. But there is usually an overlooked reason for noting that fact: we almost always learn of the technological advances after they have been achieved behind the closed doors of scientific laboratories. It was a research breakthrough enthusiastically announced by Craig Venter after the fact that escalated interest in, and worries about, synthetic biology. For security reasons, the public learned about the atom bomb only after it was developed in secret and dropped on Hiroshima. But Robert Oppenheimer, a great scientist behind the bomb, noted another feature of research: "When you see something that is technically sweet, you go ahead and do it and you argue about it only after you have had your technical success. That is the way it was with the atom bomb." In that vein, we should not forget that in the face of ethical criticism, Edwards and Steptoe simply disappeared into their laboratory in the late 1960s, releasing no information for many years on the progress of their IVF research until their announcement of the birth of baby Louise Brown in 1973. We are ultimately at the mercy and the integrity of the researchers, always playing ethical catch-up.

# 8
## Unraveling the Puzzle of Ethics

In the summer of 2009, I was attending a conference in Paris; during some free time, I took a walk along the Seine to the Musée d'Orsay. I began feeling lightheaded—so much so I had to sit down—and, once walking again, stayed near walls to lean against. I thought about getting an ambulance—well aware that the French health care system is one of the best in the world—but with classical male denial, decided to tough it out. I made the trip home, had more symptoms, finally fainted, and was rushed to a hospital diagnosed with ventricular tachycardia, a potentially lethal condition. A seven-hour "procedure" (as they called it), running a catheter up to my heart to put a laser to something or other, followed by a few week's recuperation, and altogether about $90,000 in costs, managed to save me. Along the way, I had a nice sampling of all those expensive technologies I write about, a brush with death, and the ruin of my summer vacation. I had little chance to question the need for the operation, much less shop around market-style for a better choice.

Leon R. Kass, among others, has written eloquently about the value of a finite life span in focusing our life on what is important, and many have noted the force of an impending death to fine-tune the possible insights (recall the famous line about the prospect of hanging). He may be right, but I have never felt that way. My problem has been just the opposite: how to take life seriously at the end, which can't be too far off now, when little that I might do will make any great difference in my life story. And although I found out only after my operation how close to death I had come, I had another strange reaction. When I fainted, I was out in an instant; another such episode could have killed me. But if a death of that kind, alive one minute and painlessly dead the next, were possible, it seemed to me that would be about as ideal an end that could be imagined. Had I then, with the procedure, passed up a chance for such a death? Will I better off with some other kind of death from some other kind of illness, probably much slower? That seems unlikely. Would I like a slower death to, as they say, get my affairs in order? No, they are already in order.

Asking questions of that kind, wondering whether to be saved from one kind of death by medical progress only to risk another kind—and just what counts as beneficial progress anyway—is to be forced to take a close look at the medical enterprise, rich with a mixture of benefits and burdens, joys and sorrows. For me, at least, the first and abiding question for bioethics ought to be to rethink the goals of medical research and health care delivery. But bioethics has, since its inception, accepted the status quo, the conventional goals and ends of modern enlightenment medicine. It has tried to cope with the wide range of new issues generated by them by resorting mainly to regulatory solutions (living wills, legal redefinition of death, guidelines for genetic screening), a libertarian policy with much of reproductive biology and assisted reproductive technology (ART), proceduralism for resource allocation decisions, and some variant on principlism for routine ethical problems.

## Understanding Ethics

The starting point for rethinking goals should be death itself. If death is our ultimate fate, then medicine should begin there and work its way back to the beginning of life, not forward as it now does, aiming to forestall death indefinitely. Rethinking the grand, now-sacred value of medical progress and technological innovation as its natural child are the key ingredients for a new direction in medicine and health care.

Ethics is a peculiar kind of domain. One way or the other, all of us must make moral judgments, sometimes consciously and with deliberation, at other times in an unwitting way that will reflect our personal habits, history, and cultural context. We will think hard about aggressively trying to save the life of a low-birth-weight infant with no possibility of more than a few weeks of survival—or of a severely demented elderly person who requires complex and painful treatment for survival.

But we are not likely to deliberate at all if we see a small child about to run into the street, risking our own life to save him—or inconveniently stopping on the way to an important engagement to provide CPR to a stranger lying on the street. Then there will always be some situations that do not readily have a good solution, as was the case when my mother was asked to choose between allowing her aunt to die of gangrene in her leg or have it amputated in an operation that would most likely kill her.

Ideally, we should have some orderly and rational way to manage the difficult ethical dilemmas, only some of which will have a solution satisfactory to us personally and will be reasonably persuasive to our colleagues and others whose judgment we respect. That is ethics in the formal, disciplinary sense. But then there are what we might think of as the background ethical ideals. What kind of person should I want to be, for my own sake and for those whose lives I will influence or be responsible for? In trying to answer that question, I need some insight into the way culture affects me, that of the culture of my family, my religion, my ethnic heritage, and the society in which I live.

I will have to learn in particular to distinguish my narrow self-interests and my ideological predilections given me by my personality and those background influences, and the higher ideals I should try to live by. Then I will need to have a way to put all those considerations together in some coherent way to give my life moral integrity and coherence. That effort, probably life long, is necessary both to make the conscious ethical decisions we may have to make from time to time, but no less to have those unwitting ethical habits that will make me a good person, citizen, and family member when I have no time or occasion to think things through.

Let me return here to ethical theory. I learned as a graduate student that controversy and disagreement have since the days of Plato and Aristotle marked efforts to develop a foundation of some kind for ethics. The history of moral philosophy is a history of competing theories—duty-based theories versus utilitarian consequentialist theories in particular, but both of them rejected by some for an ethic of virtue or feminist and contextualist theories—and with no resolution in sight. That struggle has been carried over into bioethics, with no resolution in sight there, either.

## Philosophy: Just What Is It All About?

Those struggles reflect the history of philosophy itself. As British philosopher John Cottingham has noted, "the last hundred years have seen an uncanny number of shifts among philosophers in their conception of what their subject is supposed to be about." Reading that sentence made me realize all over again how hard it had been to explain to my parents and in-laws just what my chosen field "is supposed to be about."

Cottingham goes on to summarize the shifts that have marked Anglo-American philosophy. It moved from a rejection of "grand theories" of reality to logical analysis (G. E. Moore, Bertrand Russell), to logical positivism (requiring all theories, ethical or otherwise, to be capable of empirical verification), to a therapeutic effort to rid philosophy of conceptual confusion (Wittgenstein), to an analysis of the structure of thought by way of an analysis of language (Michael Dummett), to a rejection of the idea of a philosopher as some kind of "cultural overseer" passing judgments on various kinds of discourse, and being reduced to narrower forms of inquiry such literature and history (Richard Rorty), to my professor at Harvard, Willard V. Quine, who espoused a science-inspired model of inquiry that should "either adopt and emulate the method of successful sciences, or . . . operate in tandem with the sciences, as their abstract and reflective branch."

The "wisdom" model of philosophy—and of moral philosophy as well—had, in this movement, disappeared in the dust. The Cottingham article appeared in a supplement of the Royal Institute of Philosophy, "Conceptions of Philosophy," in the journal *Philosophy*. Remarkably, the collection on the whole was marked by a complaint by many philosophers at the rejection of wisdom as a goal, at the aping of science, at the narrowness of the discipline, and by its embrace of a reductionistic analysis of human life and experience rather than a synthesis of their riches.

## We Can Live without Ethical Theory

Can the ideal of a moral theory be saved, and does it matter if it cannot? In answer to the second question, I would say that bioethics at least has done well enough without it. A number of fruitful ethical ideas have been brought into bioethics by physicians, theologians, social scientists, and historians, few of whom feel a need for a theoretical base. Forty years of absorption in bioethics have demonstrated to me at least that advances can be made, that many problems have been more or less solved, that presidential commissions—liberal or conservative—can say many useful and illuminating things. But note my phrase "more or less."

Every issue we took up in the 1970s is still with us, and nothing seems to get resolved once and forever with no residue. The definition of death has been affected by new scientific knowledge, as have genetic counseling and prenatal diagnosis. End-of-life care has surely moved along, but getting it just right for every dying person under whatever circumstance has proved to be as chronic a problem as the medical problems of those with chronic disease. But then most of the important issues that confront human beings, from war to crime in the streets, from the male-female relationship to having and raising children, are only "more or less" solved. And I suspect the same will be true, if we are lucky enough, with global warming and the avoidance of recessions and depressions.

## Alasdair MacIntyre and Amelie Rorty

My thinking about moral theory and its importance has been greatly shaped by the writings of the philosophers Alasdair MacIntyre and Amelie Rorty. MacIntyre's great contribution has been to show why most moral theories are incompatible and necessarily so. All of them, from Plato and Aristotle at the beginning to liberal individualism in our day, have been embedded in a particular culture and reflect the history and manifestation of that culture in the way we think. There is, most critically, no place we can stand to judge those cultures from some neutral standpoint or the ethical theories they generate. The notion of an ideal observer—and its way of distancing us from the hurly burly of human experience (as with many thought experiments)—fails to make sense in the absence of any real-world model of decision making to give it credibility.

No such view is possible, and MacIntyre is right on target to say that any view must be one from within a particular culture. The power of that culture displays itself in its ethical theories and no less so in its view of the meaning and use of reason itself. His own solution is to choose the kind of culture that gave us a Thomas Aquinas who drew upon Aristotle. But I am not sure whether we can recreate the culture and ethics of a time long past, and MacIntyre himself makes a kind of begrudging case for the liberal individualism of our culture, at least saying that it makes a certain cultural sense for us, even if in the end it is more destructive than beneficial.

Amelie Rorty's contribution is helpfully modest, yet all the stronger for that quality. Moral theories based on and aping scientific theories should be rejected as models. Instead, "we should regard them as providing leading questions, notes for consideration, pointers for critical reflection and practical deliberation . . . rather than offering competing theories, they provide prompt and direct attention to a wide variety of salient features in situations of evaluation and choice." I find this way of thinking attractive because it allows us to make use of different moral theories for different purposes in bioethics. Defining the role of the physician in the doctor-patient relationship pushes us toward virtue and duty ethics. Allocating scare resources for an entire population by legislative efforts pushes us in a utilitarian direction. No one theory can effectively take account of the different kinds of settings for moral judgment, the different kinds of moral problems that arise, and the different kinds of decisions that must be made.

## Moral Theories as Ensembles

If it is possible, then, to see moral theories as an ensemble, each capable of being used for different purposes in different contexts, and each open to combination with others, then they can be understood as a resource for ethics, not a scandal because of their diversity. Those possibilities do not of course eliminate disagreement among possible theory combinations, nor is there a method for determining how and when to combine or draw from various theories. And to talk of "theories" at all is to enter a realm high above our daily personal and professional lives. One can well ask whether at a lower, more usable, level there are some moral rules that are common in our culture and some that are universal. Various efforts have been made to find such rules, and I consider them more or less successful.

Once again I use the phrase "more or less" simply because it is usually not hard to find some groups in the United States or elsewhere who do not accept them, and there are significant differences over their application. We have come generally to believe that doctors should tell the truth to patients, following a generally acceptable moral rule that the truth should be told, but most doctors in most countries still work in a tradition of paternalism in which lying is acceptable and even considered to be necessary for patient welfare. Although I believe that doctors should tell the truth, it may be recalled that, with the collusion of her physician, we decided not to tell my mother she had cancer. But then she did not ask, either, and we judged that it would harm her to reveal the long-feared truth. In any case, it is—with many qualifications—possible to say that there is agreement that innocent people should not be killed or made to suffer, that stealing and lying are wrong, that children should be cherished and raised well, that punishment should be fair, that the elderly should be honored and their needs met, that nations should allow freedom of speech and religion, and that there should be the rule of law. Philosophers Bernard Gert, Sissela Bok, and Ruth Macklin have written persuasively on the existence of a common and universal morality. The various UN declarations of universal rights have sometimes been derided as a form of western imperialism, but—showing the power of the old saw about the tribute that vice pays to virtue—even egregious dictatorships piously pretend that they adhere to those rights.

## Ethics and Ideological Contaminants

Although I believe bioethics can do well without an underlying theory, a greater obstacle comes at the ideological level, where the conflicts reflect sharply divergent views about ways of life and primary values and can make it difficult to achieve practical agreement about particular ethical issues. They are not about formal theories of the kind that vexes philosophers, but about clusters of values and commitments that reflect different cultural and sometimes religious premises, as well as competing theories of the role of government—yet these differences are often on a continuum among the disputants.

Three examples show the tensions of ideological struggles. The Terri Schiavo case—which set off a national uproar and took years

(1990–1995) to work its way through the courts—was a struggle between the husband of Terri and her parents about whether her feeding tube that was put in place when she was diagnosed as being in a persistent vegetative state should be removed. For pro-life groups and her parents, and with the aid of some elements of the disability community, it was an effort to protect her life. For liberal groups, it was a case of following her wishes to not have the tube (or so her husband claimed). The courts eventually allowed the tube to be removed. For both groups, the case had been into one that admitted no compromise, and one for which each side had a different interpretation of the facts at stake and different notions of what it means to value life. The disability community took the position, using liberal language, that to remove her feeling tube would be an act of discrimination against a disabled person.

The national debate on the health reform legislation revealed the force of a fifty-year-old tension, clearly revealed in public opinion pools, between those inclined in market-directed reform, minimizing the government role, and those who looked to a stronger government role. The debate was pictured as a fundamental tension between individual freedom of choice and a commitment to the common good in securing coverage for the uninsured. Each side invoked deep American political and cultural values, but in a way that made it difficult to work out compromises. For both sides, more was at stake than health care. The abortion issue over the years has been for both sides no less than a clash of fundamental values as well: the status and rights of women, and the right to control one's body, over against the protection of the right to life of the innocent and the vulnerable. Yet even in that clash there were some unusual patterns: many pro-life persons, like my wife, are liberal in just about all of the rest of their politics. And there are many economic conservatives who are pro-choice on abortion.

The obvious difficulty with many bioethical problems is that they are historically new (or old ones altered by new knowledge and technologies), and that means there has not been time to work out solutions that can be called settled without residue. In at least the abortion and feeding tube cases, they are partially driven by technology, such as medically safer abortions and improved feeding tubes for the preservation of life. The health reform debate reflected the influence of the media, reflecting the in particular the influence of the social media. Telling truth to patients is still a new rule in the United States but would not be accepted at all by doctors or patients in many other countries— or by many even in our own country. Ready access to medical information on the Internet makes it harder for physicians to lie to or mislead patients. Yet the relatively recent moral rule that all patients taking part in medical research, if competent, must give their informed consent is by now a settled international moral rule. It is sometimes violated (but then what moral rule isn't?), and there remains a residue of professional arguments about what exactly the rule means, but it stands as the key rule in medical research. There are, by contrast, few settled rules about aggressive treatment of severely disabled or low-birth-weight babies, or of care at the end of life, or decisions about prostate cancer and diagnosis for those over 75 (I speak with some experience here), or whether women under the age of 50 should be routinely screened for breast cancer.

### General Rules and Discrete Individuals: The Abiding Tension

If it is a fact of some consequence that these are historically new issues that are still being worked on, it is also a fact that individuals and patients are different, requiring flexible rules and discretion and prudence in their application. If it is a good rule of public health that there need be no routine screening for breast cancer of those under age 50, it is a good rule of beneficence and physician solicitude for patient welfare that a woman with excessive anxieties about breast cancer be an exception to the rule. The greatest good of the greatest number is a fine principle for public health policy (quarantines can be imposed), but all the better if complemented by a rule of physician and patient discretion in some circumstances; however, it may not be easy to specify those circumstances with any firm rules. In ethics, as in much of the rest of our lives, there will always be a final gap, sometime large and sometimes small, between our rules, principles, and theories and actual decision making. This is true whether the domain is foreign policy, international trade agreements, stimulus packages for a recession, just when to get out of Afghanistan— and bioethics.

I have dropped along the way in this book a variety of hints, and sometimes outright efforts to proselytize a different point of view, about how I think ethics is best understood and examined. It is a view far more untidy than most philosophers will tolerate. I am a philosopher by training, but not one in the way I think, which is much more interdisciplinary. The seeds of this difference were planted in my courses in college; my embrace of a broad and probably too romantic a vision of philosophy inspired by the life and dialogs of Socrates; my repugnance at the way ethics was conceptualized and taught at Harvard, as well as the narrowness of philosophy more generally; my work as an editor of *Commonweal*, writing for an educated public; my perception that ethics is something that is grasped by everyone; the difference between ethicists on and off duty; the role of passion, interests, and ideology underneath ostensibly rational, neutral ways of thinking; and, through my work in health policy, the need for a new way of thinking about the ethical ends and means of the medical enterprise itself.

A good deal of my own biases creep in here—sometimes, I suppose, more a matter of taste and temperament than of ethical substance. If I were a painter, I would paint murals in splashy colors, not well-crafted miniatures. My reading of good literature, where the prose flows and pulls one along, has made me restless when I read sentences in philosophy and ethics that have to be read a number of times to understand (as one contributor to the Royal Society collection has complained about as well). My own efforts at wisdom, not notably successful or improved by aging, have convinced me there is no royal road to that goal. One of the wisest of all books on ethics was by theologian Langdon Gilkey: *Shantung Compound*, which is about how he and his fellow prisoners in a WWII Japanese prisoner worked out among themselves how to live with each other in the face of fear, cruelty, and deprivation. If I were teaching bioethics, which I won't ever do again, I would make Gilkey's book, Richard Rhodes's *The Making of the Atom Bomb*, some Socratic dialogs, and Tolstoy's story *The Death of Ivan Ilyich* required reading, with Dubos, Rieff, and Christopher Lasch as chasers. That is, with the exception of the Tolstoy story, I would not start with readings in bioethics at all. As with physical exercise, bioethics should begin with some warm-up exercises, a flexing and loosening of the mental muscles—what we called "cross-training" when I was swimming: using different muscles with different strokes.

## The Influence of Culture

One likely reason I have not been drawn to doing bioethics in the traditional disciplinary style is that my interest in medicine and bioethics has been greatly influenced by a fascination with the culture of American medicine, requiring different skills and knowledge to understand. The United States is idiosyncratic in taking so long to get universal care (and still will not cover everyone), in resisting price controls on drugs and devices, in its mixture of private and government-financed coverage, in the high fees and salaries paid to physicians, and its failure to control costs. But the culture of American medicine shows that it is the offspring of American culture and, not coincidentally, the most dedicated to medical research and technological innovation. Our health care system is as good an instance of (sometimes derided) "American exceptionalism" as one can find.

Let me look at three great changes in the social impact of medical developments in recent decades and how they were in turn nurtured by the background national culture: changing conceptions of medicine, of health, and of living a life. Other than post–World War II affluence, it is hard to think of any scientific developments that have had an equally profound effect on our national life.

American medicine is the most complicated in the world, replete with superb physicians and medical centers but also full of regional variations and inequities and high costs—and with health outcomes that have long lagged behind those of other developed countries. Its most distinctive feature is the unique relationship among the market, affluence, and technological innovation. As good a symbol of that relationship is the National Institutes of Health, the leading biomedical research center in the world. The pharmaceutical and device industries directly gain from NIH's basic research and are among the largest and most profitable of industries. American physicians are the highest paid in the world, with a dominance of subspecialty physicians who command the highest fees. American medical students have overwhelmingly gone into those specialties in recent years in order to pay medical school debts but also because their income will be more than if they went into primary care.

It is no accident that fee-for-service is the most common form of physician reimbursement, paying more for the use of technology than talking with patients. Most, but hardly all, physicians seem to like it that way. Nor is it an accident that the Medicare program does not allow its administrators to take costs into account in determining its benefits. Some groups of physicians also like it that way, and the medical industries have lobbied for years to make sure that policy is not changed. Again and again the health care industry, on the delivery and research side, trumpets its central importance in the American economy, lately underscored by health care as one of the industries that has added jobs to the economy in the face of recession.

### The Troubled Marriage of Commerce and Medicine

American medicine and the health care system of which it is a part are heavily commercial in their values and aspirations. In its love of progress, medicine is hardly distinguishable from other industries dependent on technological innovation for growth and economic competitiveness. It is something of a miracle that most physicians remain faithful to their professional values in a system that does all it can to turn them into better businessmen, which in fact they must be to fit into the health care system. But that is not altogether new. Plato once spoke of the doctor as a "business man."

If medicine itself has changed over the recent decades, so has the public and professional understanding of health. It was at one time possible to think of health simply as the proper working of the body and mind. Medicine's aim was to thwart illness and disease, to restore lost function, and to care for those who could not be cured. Death was accepted as inevitable. At some point in the twentieth century—I would say by the 1960s—medicine entered a more messianic phase.

What I have called the great schism in medicine began to appear: a tension between medicine's traditional mission of caring for the sick and its newfound power to save life, and to treat death itself as a kind of biological accident—one that would, by steadily vanquishing lethal diseases one by one, gradually fade away. The medicalization of our lives has been a rich area for sociologists and anthropologists. There is no fatal disease that the NIH is not out to conquer. Its annual plea to Congress is: give us more research money and we will eventually do so.

Put another way, at the same time that the hospice and palliative care movements were emerging in the late 1960s and early 1970s to restore medicine to its ancient role of caring for the dying, the research side was stepping up its war against disease and death, ever more confident of success. Old-time fatalism was rejected, and the kind of traditional hope that physicians were taught to instill in their patients even in the face of death has now been transferred to the research side of medicine: don't despair, relief is on the way. "Rage, rage, against the dying of the light" might well be adopted as the NIH's favorite line of poetry. The chronic difficulty I have earlier mentioned with end-of-life care stems in great part from the hope and hype coming from a messianic research agenda that has erased any bright line between living and dying and instills instead a too-common belief among patients in medical miracles, which physicians now complain about.

That transformation in thinking about health itself as far more open to change and radical improvement found some uniquely American support in the media. With the possible exception of the United Kingdom, the coverage of news about medical treatments and progress is enormous. "Promising" new breakthroughs, particularly on cancer and Alzheimer's disease, are almost weekly stories. One has to read to the very end of the articles to find the all-too-frequent qualifications that the research was on mice and that it could be years before it reaches the public, if ever. Stories of that kind are matched by pieces about maintaining one's personal health through diet, exercise, advice on medical screening, and, when all else fails, the possibilities of cosmetic surgery to make one at least look younger and healthier. The media particularly projects a tacit belief that it is not the body that necessarily fails but that the failure can, retrospectively, be traced to a lack of good medical care, poor health-related behavior, underused and inadequate medical screening, and does so prospectively, by breathlessly hawking the notion that technology-driven cures are just around the corner. All of these features of American health care are greatly enhanced by the medical and drug industries, which push their products relentlessly with physicians and hospitals and by direct-to-consumer advertising. It's not just about health care as a right, but that idea has been escalated to a right to good health.

We have yet to learn how to properly assess new medical technologies for their economic, individual, and social impact. As matters now stand, it is difficult to do so. Industry has its own reasons for resisting a prior economic assessment of its products. Many physicians worry about an interference with the doctor-patient relationship with comparative and cost-effectiveness research. Researchers at the basic science level do not want to be hampered by heavy ethical scrutiny or a demanding risk-benefit analysis. The net result is that it is nearly impossible to stop upstream research, particularly in the private sector, which—once loosed on society—is often difficult to control and regulate. The ART industry is a good instance of a wide range of problems stemming from a lack of oversight and regulation.

There is some worry about the potential dangers of synthetic biology research and applications, but they are easily warded off by focusing on the potential benefits, not harms. As any number of efforts to assess new technologies have shown, it is standard practice for their inventors and supporters to make a strong, usually excessive, case for the benefits and portray opposition as ethical hand-wringing or Ludditism. A colleague of mine was asked after his presentation at a congressional hearing on synthetic biology what he thought of the proceedings. It was designed, he felt, as an occasion to trumpet the wonderful possible benefits of the research and to minimize the hazards. It was, he said, "congressional theater." The President's Council that did a study of it concluded in the conventional way that there are benefits and dangers but that the latter could be taken care of by some cautious oversight.

## Bioethics as Loyal Dissent

I have always thought that bioethics should be a loyal dissenter in the onward march of medical progress, loyal because it can do us good, but needing dissent because it has the capacity to carry us away in utopian reveries and ill-considered actions. It is one of those things in modern life one cannot live with or live without. Put more precisely, we cannot live well without paying a price for it, and not live well if we don't know when to use it. The conservative President's Council on Bioethics had the nerve to raise some basic questions about the medical enterprise and to try relating them to some ancient knowledge and insight. Its shrewd choice of Hawthorne's tale "The Birthmark" for its opening discussion was just right in my eyes. It was just wrong in the eyes of its liberal critics, failing to jump right in on pressing policy issues.

As it happened, I had resigned some twenty-five years earlier from the New York Council on Life and Law—aiming for a state confrontation with bioethics—when Governor Mario Cuomo said that it should aim to produce policy recommendations for the legislature. I argued that public education was a far more important goal. The major failing of the President's Council was not in evading policy issues, which it actually did not, but in staying far away from the role of industry and market values in paying for many of the things that it wanted our society to resist.

The failure of the liberal councils, which made many useful policy recommendations, was that they shied away from just those deeper questions that liberal individualism and secular division find too troubling, for the most part, to be discussed at all. I do not think that was a conscious decision: it goes with the territory of shaping policy. But it almost inevitably ends up playing handmaiden to industry, the research enterprise, and to an all-too-common libertarianism that supports individual choice, whatever the choice. Too often, it ends by polishing the ethical means of the American medical and health enterprise at the expense of the ethical ends. About the only time it raises its voice is to complain that justice in the allocation of the goodies of progress is being rationed. The goodies themselves are rarely questioned, and when they are, the price to be paid is to be called (gulp) a conservative by liberals and a do-good liberal by conservatives. Bush's council, by ignoring the role of the governance and the market as often enough enemies of morality, had a parallel failing.

Just how bioethics should best make its contribution to medicine and health care can itself be seen as an ethical dilemma: that of finding a good balance between helping them with ethical insights and useful clinical and policy analysis, and standing outside and apart ready to call them to moral account. That problem has never been solved, and my own conviction is obvious, but it is crucial to solve it to keep the field alive and well. Sometimes the ends of medicine, and the commercial and research interests that nourish it, need to be questioned. Above all else, our field should "speak truth to power" (to use the late Adam Wildavsky's pungent phrase).

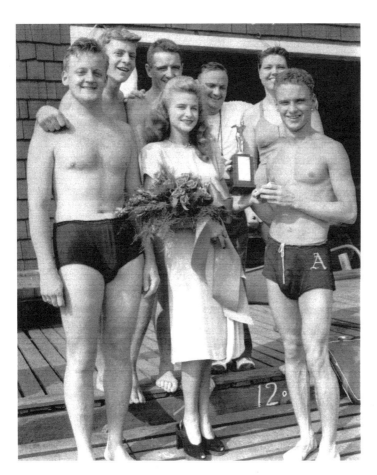

**Figure 1**
Washington, D.C., long-distance swimming champion Daniel Callahan with Ms.
Washington, D.C. 1948.

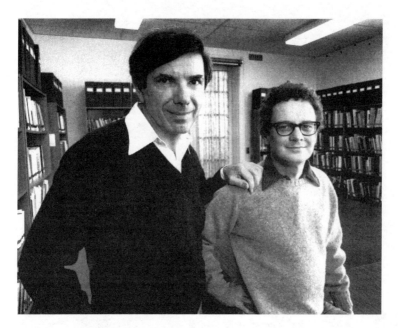

**Figure 2**
Daniel Callahan and Willard Gaylin, cofounders of the Hastings Center, 1973.

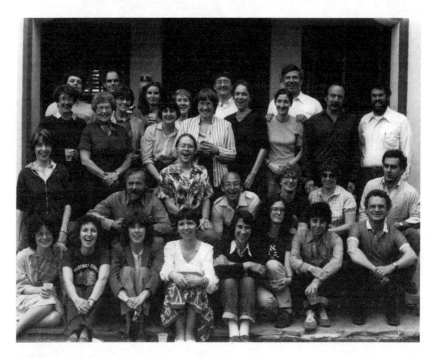

**Figure 3**
Hastings Center staff and visiting scholars, 1981.

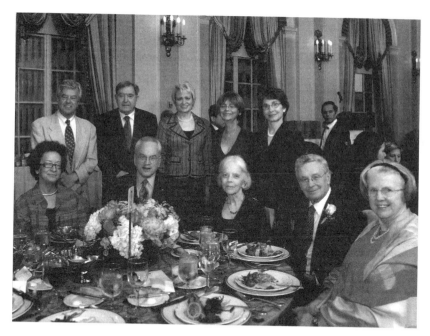

**Figure 4**

Fortieth anniversary of the Hastings Center. Back row, from left: Tom Beauchamp; Arnold S. Relman, editor emeritus, *New England Journal of Medicine*; Susan Dentzler, editor-in-chief, *Health Affairs*; Ruth Faden, Johns Hopkins Medical School; Marcia Angell, editor emeritus, *New England Journal of Medicine*. Front row, from left: Irene Crow, Pettus-Crow Foundation; Mark Callahan, New York University; Sidney Callahan; Daniel Callahan; Sissela Bok.

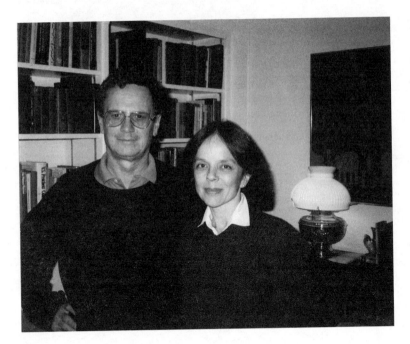

**Figure 5**
Sidney and Daniel Callahan, 1987.

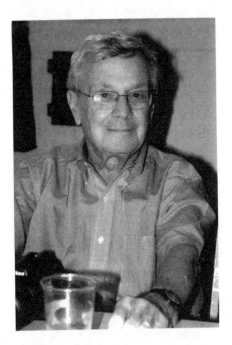

**Figure 6**
Daniel Callahan, 2010.

# 9
## Reaching the Finish Line

Until not long ago, I believed that I had been born during one of the best eras of America history and that the timing of my birth was a bit of added benefit. Now I am not so sure. I came into the world just as the Great Depression was beginning to, but into a family that was not affected by it. I was too young to be drafted during WWII and too old for the Vietnam War. I was the right age for the Korean War but did my service under one of the oddest, least life-threatening, circumstances: living at home with my parents and commuting to the Pentagon looking for desks that were not locked or safes that were left open.

My wife and I had our children during the baby boom period, which turned out to the most prosperous of the twentieth century. During the mid-1960s, Senator Daniel Patrick Moynihan told me that the main problem facing the federal government was that "it had too much money to spend and did not know how to spend it." I helped start the Center at a time when money was still available to create a research center—even for someone with six children and no job, and whose children could to go to college without taking out any loans. Save for my emphysema and a heart operation (routine afflictions at my age), I reached my 80s in good shape. The Center celebrated my 80th birthday with a wonderful party and the publication of a booklet collecting many of the articles I had written for the *Hastings Center Report*: "The Daniel Callahan Reader."

As it has turned out, the final years of my life have seen a bad, extended recession, not nearly as dangerous as that of the Great Depression but enough to make almost everyone anxious and with millions in or facing poverty. In some ways the worst part of it has been the political scene, one marked by ideological gridlock, a nasty bipartisan rhetoric, and a growing sense that not only our democracy itself is threatened but our entire way of life.

At its bottom, the political debate is about a clash of values, and those, I have come to think, are the worst kind to deal with. I got my first taste of that in working on the abortion problem, one that to this day shows no sign of compromise or reconciliation, pitting pro-life against pro-choice adversaries. During the early years of the Center, there were some who said that given the ambivalence and skepticism the word "ethics" seemed to provoke in medical circles, we should instead present our work as focusing on "values," a softer, less hazardous word. Someone once made that case by noting, with a touch of irony, that by deliberately casting ethical problems in the language of values the BBC was able to avoid controversy.

We were not persuaded to make that change, but the issue came up again at the Center in 2009 when we published a fine collection of papers on "Connecting American Values with Health Reform." The aim was to see whether we could bring to the reform debate a different way of framing the policy issues, drawing on a variety of values common in our history and culture. It was a collection that got a positive reception in Washington, seeming to have the anodyne effect we intended; it went down smoothly and uncontroversially. Yet as time went on, I began to realize that the language of values was itself part of the problem, working against a resolution of the reform conflicts. The trouble was that the worst conflicts are themselves conflicts over basic values ("here I stand"): individual good versus common good; government regulation versus consumer choice; justice versus individual rights, and so on—long-standing struggles in American life. They often turn out to be hostile to compromise if used by single-minded ideological adversaries or as rhetorical flourishes to prove one's patriotic credentials. Could it be, I wondered, if the best thing that could happen politically would be the disappearance of fiercely held values? When fundamental values are in conflict, there are no ways using the language of values to resolve them.

But if the language of values turned out to be a false or at least unhelpful friend in Washington, that may be even more true of the word "ethics." It soon became clear that the dominant intellectual disciplines in the Washington political debates are those of economics and the technical policy disciplines, occasionally now and then political science, especially if empirically oriented. The word "ethics" either draws no response at all or, even more likely, is seen to offer nothing as a formal discipline or a fruitful way of talking about public policy—sometimes, it seems, even feared as itself a source of unresolvable conflicts or a weapon that can be used to tarnish reputations and blacken policy positions as immoral.

The most conspicuous evidence of this was the terror, shared by both parties, of any discussion of rationing. We learned this the hard way when we proposed to one prominent and influential Washington policy center, the Bipartisan Policy Center—which had solicited our help—that we do some work on ethical means of rationing, particularly in the certain event that Medicare benefits would have to be cut. Although I can't prove it, the fact is that we were abruptly dropped by them once we made that proposal. Only later did we learn that there is full bipartisan agreement that the word "rationing" is utterly unacceptable in Washington. Sarah Palin's greatest triumph was coming up with the phrase "death panels," effective not only in scaring everyone away from the word rationing but also in closing the door to the likely need for some kind of committee to make Medicare rationing decisions. I might note, however, that a number of articles have appeared in leading medical and policy journals over the past few years talking directly about, and using the word, "rationing." That makes the allergy to it in Washington seem all the striking—the one place in a position to actually do it.

In any event, even beyond that issue, bioethics has had no role of any consequence in the reform debate. A number of us wrote articles and blogs on one or more reform topics, but mainly in the professional literature. Hardly any of us were invited to take part in the almost weekly conferences or panels put together by the numerous researchers centers in Washington. I had no good evidence at all that my health care cost monitor blog had any impact whatsoever in Washington despite it having been called one of the most valuable of all health care blogs.

By the end of 2011, my energy for health care issues debates had run down. They were both fascinating and stimulating for a time but eventually became repetitive, the congressional stalemates almost depressing. The health care reform act was a major victory for the President Obama and the Democrats and is even now taking effect. But it has some major

Republican obstruction ahead of it, the possibility of a Republican president and Republican Congress in the coming election, and mixed public support. It is impossible to guess how it will all work out, particularly now that it has become ensnared in the still larger, even more acrid argument about reducing the national debt.

As it happened, it was that debate which led me in a new direction in 2011. I organized a project entitled "Assessing National Priorities." I had observed time and time again how often medical and policy journals, and the media, noted that health care costs were crowding out other national needs at both the national and state levels. Health care expenditures were about 6 percent of the GDP forty years ago, and defense and education about 5 percent each. By 2011, health care costs were 18 percent of the GDP, defense and education around 4.5 percent, and education slightly over 5 percent. Health care costs have far outrun the others, with the Medicaid program creating particularly heavy pressures at the state level.

A useful exercise would be to pursue this question: apart from money, how should national priorities be assessed, and what might they best be? It turned out to be a devilishly hard project, attempting to find ways of comparing like with unlike needs: defense versus education; education versus health care; environment versus space exploration; public parks versus early childhood education; economic security in old age versus job security—and then to see if it would be possible to propose a rank order for all of them (and there are other categories as well).

Much to our surprise, we could not find any previous efforts to do that sort of thing. The word "priorities" is often used in policy literature, but most efforts simply set the different national needs side by side without actually proposing priorities, much less rank ordering them. The most obvious difficulty in doing so is finding some kind of common metric that can be used with all the needs. We were never able to discover such a thing or devise one ourselves—at least not one with any decisive clout to make the necessary comparisons. Fortunately, however, a strong movement is afoot among economists and others to move away from using the GDP and its growth as the main measure of national welfare. If nothing else, the economic growth of the GDP provides no clue as to the fair distribution of the wealth that might come from it. A major study commissioned in 2008 by President Sarkozy of France,

"Commission on the Measurement of Economic Performance and Social Progress," chaired by two Nobel laureates—Joseph Stiglitz and Amartya Sen—worked to develop criteria for national well-being other than an economic one. At the same time, a number of what have been called social indicators studies or sometimes happiness studies were setting out to determine exactly what social conditions are most productive of overall human welfare.

We decided in the end to present some alternative scenarios of America's future. One of them would be to continue pursuing the role that fell to (or was grasped by) the United States after World War II, that of maintaining the world's strongest economy and most powerful military force. A second would be to seriously lower those international aspirations and to pursue instead improvements in the quality and fairness of our common domestic life. We now rank first in economy and defense but are far down the comparative list versus other countries on the quality of our life. The priority of the former should decline and the latter increase. A third scenario would be to find some middle way between those two possibilities. The project has been difficult but uncommonly rewarding, forcing everyone who is a part of it to become familiar with just about everything about American society and its values and to determine how the ensemble of our national needs and desires can be made sense of and ordered (at least on paper) in the wisest way.

As if that project were not enough to keep me busy, I began writing a new book entitled, "The Five Horsemen: Managing Global Crises." I had long and in a most amateurish way followed the debate on global warming and the threat it poses to our globe and everyone on it. I was constantly struck by the parallels between efforts to reduce that warming and our health care reform efforts. Both are far from a good solution, the situation for both is worsening not improving, both find both public and commercial resistance to real change, and both are weighed down by scientific controversies and competing ideas for dealing with them. As I thought more about it, I noticed four other international crises that if, not exactly identical, have some significant family resemblances to the global warming and health care debates (and some interesting overlaps as well): clean water and drought, food shortages, obesity, and chronic illness.

Drought and food shortages are in part caused by climate change, but require their own policy strategies. Obesity is a major cause of chronic illness, but each has to be approached differently. Population growth and aging societies, two of my earliest interests, come into play as well.

Yet even as I was starting that book, I found something missing from those large-scale international problems and debates that I had come to cherish with ethics and health care, subjects I could intimately connect with my own life. I know what it is like to get sick and to hurt, just as I know what it is to have family members and friends die. I have no direct experience with global warming or with drought and food shortages, or obesity (but some with chronic illness). This was brought home to me when I had to set aside work on the global crises to write a paper for a conference on care at the end of life—and how different it is to think about that issue.

I must have written at least four articles already on that topic over the past decade, and each of them could have had the same title: "Care at the End of Life: Why Has It Been So Hard?" My literary vanity will not allow me to keep using that title: even if it has the same content, the unwritten rule among repetitive writers is that each article must have a new title. The latest title was "Care at the End of Life: A Philosophical or Management Problem?" It is not hard to guess how I answered that question. But it is a topic I could not stay away from. I cannot fail to note how it brings together so many threads of my ethical thinking— and, not irrelevantly, a topic not wholly academic for someone my age. It has everything someone of my calling could ask for: death, aging, moral decisions, medical uncertainty, industry and the play of the market, the rise of chronic disease, patient and physician confusion and ambivalence, technological wizardry, and a steady stream of stories, personal and in the media, about care at the end of life that is wonderful or outrageously bad, and about the lives of patients that ended terribly or touchingly or their family caretakers who were edified by the experience or nearly destroyed by it. It is, in other words, an issue that brings together in one great Gordian knot almost all that is good and bad about American medicine and health care, which still awaits an emperor to slice through it.

No, that last metaphor is not right. Despite all the grand solutions I have offered over the years, matched only by a few hundred offered by others, it is a knot that will not be sliced, but can only be frayed. Slices have been made in the knot by advances in palliative care, by a powerful and still growing hospice movement (now caring for some 1 million patients a year, but too many coming to it too late), by a more educated public on their options in their dying, and by more doctors trained to better care for the terminally ill. But although it was one of the first research topics taken up by the Hastings Center in the 1970s, the problem just does not go away and, if anything, may be harder and more complex now.

It often seems harder now because, after some forty years of medical progress, there are more effective ways to keep sick people alive longer, more ways to save more organs, and more complicated choices to be offered to patients and families. It has become harder, not easier, to find a bright line between living and dying, between patients who can (might, could, possibly) be saved and those whose situation is, as they used to say, hopeless. Technological possibilities blur all lines. Then there is that good old standby, the technological imperative—often condemned but never vanquished—which holds that what can be done for patients ought to be done. It is matched by the research imperative with its multipronged war on death, its continuing bulletins from the front that fatalism is no longer acceptable, that if death itself cannot be defeated, then everything that causes it can be. That message has been heard by patients: however bleak the prognosis, it just might apply in their case.

But the enduring difficulty is that, as human beings, our will to live is strong, not easily overcome. I have been able to persuade a few people that it is good for the vitality of the species that we all die and be replaced by a younger generation. But that does not mean, even for true species-loving believers, that it is good for them as individuals, that their lives (unless they are utterly and irredeemably miserable) are the better for dying. At the least, it deprives us of the love and presence of others, something death can in no way compensate us for. The hope for life that modern medicine simultaneously feeds upon and nourishes, the promising new treatments always coming along, and the doctors trained to save us and the families that don't want to lose us make the downward slope of a peaceful death come to look more like an uphill climb to actually bring it about.

## Ethics and Medicine: Art and Science

The first lesson I learned about medicine as the Center was getting underway is that it is an uncertain science and a difficult art. That perception was in a way a comfort for someone like me, railed at on occasion by doctors asserting that we philosophers and other so-called bioethical experts have many questions and few answers. Care at the end of life is an exercise in medical and ethical uncertainty, with many questions and few answers. Or, better put, there are many good answers but not quite enough, and we have to drop some that do not work out. Our ethical answers can suffer the same fate. The aim should not be certainty, elusive at best, but the more modest goal of walking through the dense underbrush, looking for some good paths and learning to watch out for brambles. We will get somewhere, even if we don't know now where that will be.

In the meantime, I think of my children's future now that they have already reached middle age. I worry about the outcome of the health care and deficit debates and how it will affect their health care and economic security in their old age. I worry no less about the political and economic future of the country, and whether and in what ways it will hold together. And will the oceans have risen, the droughts be more widespread, the water shortages more devastating, and obesity and chronic disease still be with us?

"Crib death," the condition that killed my newborn baby Thomas after 42 days of life, is still not understood. Middle age was not in his future. My daughter Sarah has persistent and severe back pains that have not been fully diagnosed or adequately treated despite the attention of many specialists. She has been drawn to alternative medicine, which often happens when conventional medicine is failing. Her younger son has Tourette's syndrome, a misery for which no cure has been found, but it may go away when he gets older. My son John has had three successful knee operations, occasioned by his unwillingness at age 50 to give up amateur soccer. (I can recall vividly a conversation with a group of doctors in the early 1970s scoffing at the desire of a tennis player to have medicine cure his tennis elbow, saying, "You are 40 years old, get over it.") My son Mark, the oldest, is in otherwise good health but says he finds it hard to accept a decline in his energy (which I know all about).

My son David and his wife Wendy recently lamented the fact that their son, Alexander, conceived via IVF, would not have a sibling. Their spare frozen embryo did not take. Peter is also healthy, save for some perennial anxiety, which is well managed with medications. Stephen has long had some fairly severe asthma problems, and we share similar breathing (or nonbreathing) experiences.

In sum, save for Thomas, they have all made their way into middle age in reasonably good shape, with few serious problems along the way. Because all of them were born between 1955 and 1965, they personify the baby boom generation—just the group my Medicare writings have focused on. I try to imagine what their lives will be like thirty years from now, roughly the gap that separates my present age from theirs. That is an even harder exercise with my five grandchildren. What life will be like sixty-five or seventy-five years from now is even more opaque. But then my mother, born in 1895, could hardly have imagined at the end of the nineteenth century what life would be like when she died in 1981.

In a Dutch cemetery in the neighboring town of Tarrytown, there is a 1685 tombstone with the names of five children on it, all of whom died in the space of one week, no doubt from some epidemic, and not a few graves of young women who died in childbirth. We have been spared those kinds of disaster, but they are still a reality in many poor countries. It has been more than a blessing for us that most of our children survived. I can praise medical progress, with the help of affluence, for that. Whether that continuing progress will be good or bad for them as they move into old age is a story yet to be told.

# Index

## Basic Bioethics

Arthur Caplan, editor

## Books Acquired under the Editorship of Glenn McGee and Arthur Caplan

Karen F. Greif and Jon F. Merz, *Current Controversies in the Biological Sciences: Case Studies of Policy Challenges from New Technologies*

Deborah Blizzard, *Looking Within: A Sociocultural Examination of Fetoscopy*

Ronald Cole-Turner, ed., *Design and Destiny: Jewish and Christian Perspectives on Human Germline Modification*

Holly Fernandez Lynch, *Conflicts of Conscience in Health Care: An Institutional Compromise*

Mark A. Bedau and Emily C. Parke, eds., *The Ethics of Protocells: Moral and Social Implications of Creating Life in the Laboratory*

Jonathan D. Moreno and Sam Berger, eds., *Progress in Bioethics: Science, Policy, and Politics*

Eric Racine, *Pragmatic Neuroethics: Improving Understanding and Treatment of the Mind-Brain*

Martha J. Farah, ed., *Neuroethics: An Introduction with Readings*

Jeremy R. Garrett, ed., *The Ethics of Animal Research: Exploring the Controversy*

## Books Acquired under the Editorship of Arthur Caplan

Sheila Jasanoff, ed., *Reframing Rights: Bioconstitutionalism in the Genetic Age*

Christine Overall, *Why Have Children? The Ethical Debate*

Yechiel Michael Barilan, *Human Dignity, Human Rights, and Responsibility: The New Language of Global Bioethics and Bio-Law*

Tom Koch, *Thieves of Virtue: When Bioethics Stole Medicine*

Timothy F. Murphy, *Ethics, Sexual Orientation, and Choices about Children*

Daniel Callahan, *In Search of the Good: A Life in Bioethics*